Tissue Engineering for Neonatal Congenital Heart Disease: A New Frontier in Pediatric Cardiac Care

Ambrose

First Printing, 2024

Table of Contents

Chapter 1. Introduction and Background

1. Congenital Heart Disease and the Fontan Procedure

The field of tissue engineering represents a rapidly progressing discipline which provides new tools for surgeons and clinicians to manage complex clinical diseases. A hallmark of tissue engineering, the ability of new autologous tissues that can integrate into the host, has provided unique solutions to treating neonatal congenital heart disease (CHD). While treatment has improved over time, neonatal CHD is still a pressing clinical concern with

1-2% of newborns suffering from CHD. CHD also remains the primary cause of birth defect-related deaths in newborns [1-3]. Surgical based interventions remain a pillar of care with ~25% of CHD patients requiring surgery in the first year of life [4, 5]. Prenatal diagnosis of CHD newborns that will require surgery continues to improve as well. From 2006 to 2012, the prenatal diagnosis rate of CHD patients that would require surgery within the first 6 months of life increased from 26% to 42%, representing improved surgical planning capabilities [6]. With the improved surgical intervention and the survival of neonates/infants with CHD into adulthood reaching 90%, the rate of reoperation continues to rise as well [7-9]. Reoperation in CHD patients brings additional challenges such as increased surgical complications from pericardial adhesions and increased associated mortality [10-14]. These downstream associated risks necessitate careful surgical planning and management of CHD early in a neonate's life. In this capacity, tissue engineering provides novel approaches to CHD surgical interventions, addressing the limitations of current implantable materials, such as restricted growth, risk for thrombosis, infection, and limited endothelialization [15-18].

Surgical management of various CHD malformations can be categorized as either palliative or curative, with the need for new tissue dependent upon the specific surgical approach. The most prevalent, serious congenital heart malformations that necessitate surgery include hypoplastic left heart syndrome (HLHS), tetralogy of Fallot (TOF), tricuspid valve atresia, and transposition of the great arteries. HLHS is a sequela of left-sided defects including aortic valve and mitral valve stenosis or atresia, an underdeveloped or non-existent left ventricle, and underdevelopment of the aortic arch / aorta (**Figure 1-1**) [19]. The failed development of the left side of the heart necessitates dependence on the right side to supply circulation through the ductus arteriosus [20]. Without surgical intervention, prognosis is almost inevitability fatal [21, 22]. The standard surgical management of HLHS is a three-stage palliative surgical approach beginning with the Norwood procedure and ending in a Fontan procedure, allowing blood to bypass the ventricles and travel directly to the lungs (**Figure 1-1**) [23].

The first stage of the procedure, the Norwood or similar variations, is performed within the first few days after birth. It creates a temporary Blalok-Taussig shunt between the subclavian artery and the pulmonary veins and utilizes patches to repair defects in the aorta as well as in atrial and ventricular walls. The second stage, commonly referred to as a bidirectional Glenn or hemi-Fontan procedure, is performed around six months of age. In this procedure the superior vena cava is disconnected from the right atrium and anastomosed to the pulmonary arteries. Finally, the Fontan, performed at 1.5-3 years of age, disconnects the inferior vena cava from the right atrium and connects it to the pulmonary artery by utilizing a graft for the unavailable vessel length, completing the single ventricle conversion [23].

The Fontan procedure can be further separated into either a lateral tunnel Fontan or an extracardiac Fontan approach with both ultimately connecting the IVC to pulmonary artery [24]. The lateral tunnel method involves utilizing the now unused atrium as a conduit between the native inferior vena cava and the pulmonary arteries, typically also utilizing an additional graft material to complete the full wall of the graft. The extracardiac Fontan relies on non-autologous materials for creating the conduit that utilize either synthetic ePTFE (Gore-Tex) or donor tissue such as aortic homograft [24, 25]. The use of synthetic materials poses additional challenges to short-term and long-term surgical success. In the first-stage palliative care for HLHS, aortic arch reconstruction with synthetic or donor tissue suffers from rapid outgrowing by the patient [26].

In addition to HLHS, the Fontan procedure is utilized as palliative management of tricuspid atresia. All pre-surgical medical treatment for these patients focuses on management until a Fontan can be performed [27-29].

While advancement in the surgical techniques and clinical management of neonatal CHD has allowed more neonates to reach adulthood, the long-term success remains unclear. A recent large-scale report of post-Fontan patient follow-up found 90% survival at 30 years of age and 80% survival at 40 years of age. However, the majority (59%) had serious complications with 21% requiring re-operation [30]. Another report found the incidence of heart failure post-Fontan for single ventricle repair to be 40% [31]. In the Fontan procedure, the extracardiac Fontan continues to grow in popularity as the preferred approach due to advantages such as its applicability to a broad spectrum of anatomic presentations and amenability in a heart transplant procedure [32, 33]. This technique's rise in use brings with it a greater necessity for donor tissue and/or material to form the conduit; however, concerns over the increased risk of thrombosis and stenosis by using a conduit remain. Non-synthetic donor tissue includes autologous pericardium, bovine xenografts, and homografts [34-40]. While these options pose some advantages, such as the potential for luminal endothelialization seen in pedicled pericardium, they ultimately face disadvantages due to limited donor tissue availability and the risk of venous thrombosis as seen in the bovine xenografts [36, 41-43]. Dacron and Gore-Tex (ePTFE) synthetic conduits pose a viable alternative due to ease of availability, but additionally face challenges. Dacron grafts used in the extracardiac Fontan result in a high rate of stenosis [44]. Gore-Tex conduits face their own challenge of patient somatic overgrowth leading to surgical delay in the newborn until the IVC has approached a diameter closer to that of its final adult size [45-47]. Tissue engineered vascular grafts (TEVGs) address the limitations faced by other implantable materials in the extracardiac Fontan by being readily available, patient specific, thrombosis resistant, and capable of growth [48].

While the long-term survival of TOF patients has been shown to reach 92% at 20 years, the percent of these survivors requiring reoperation is around 53% [49]. Notably, the majority of post corrective TOF patients will experience pulmonary regurgitation at 5-10 years post-surgical management. Pulmonary valve replacement thus represents a common follow-up intervention with 36% to 40% of surviving TOF patients requiring it [50, 51]. Concern over pulmonary valve replacement occurring too late in TOF patients to be beneficial necessitates re-evaluation of intervention earlier after corrective TOF surgery [52]. The obvious consequence of this is questions over the longevity of pulmonary valve replacements and complications that can arise over a patient's life. Surgical based pulmonary valve replacement in TOF patients has shown moderate success. Mechanical and homograft replacement valves have been shown to have 10-year re-operation free rate among survivors of 87% (mechanical) and 74% to 89% (homograft) [53-55]. Longer term follow-up to determine the longevity of these valve replacements in aging TOF patients remains to be determined.

2. Tissue Engineering Topical Overview

As described above, outcomes of current surgical procedures used in congenital heart diseases are limited by the use of prosthetic materials used to create replacement heart valves, vascular grafts, and cardiopulmonary patches. Use of these materials is often complicated by limited durability and the risks of infection, host immune response, and thrombotic complications. The lack of growth and remodeling potential is also a particularly hazardous limitation in the case of pediatric patients. The field of tissue engineering holds promise for surgical solutions for these patients that can rise above these issues.

Tissue engineering, first described as a field by Langer and Vacanti in 1993, promotes the idea of using the body's natural growth and regeneration processes to repair and replace damaged and nonfunctioning organs with healthy, native tissue [56]. Many approaches exist within tissue engineering, including the use of biodegradable polymeric scaffolds, decellularized extracellular matrix, stem cells, and harvested patient cells [57]. Each of these techniques has had its own successes, and each is characterized by its own set of limitations.

The environment in which the construct grows will influence the histological structure and extracellular matrix formed [58]. Researchers have approached this phenomenon from several perspectives. In one approach, the formation of tissue begins *in vitro* by seeding cells onto a biodegradable scaffold and then maturing the tissue in a bioreactor prior to implantation *in vivo*. Using this approach, the scaffold is used as a cell delivery system and implanted *in vivo* shortly after cell attachment has taken place [59]. This approach uses a cell-scaffold construct to provide the initial structural integrity necessary to provide temporary physiological function until neotissue grows and remodels. The technique proposes that appropriate environmental signals for tissue repair and remodeling are inherently present in the *in vivo* milieu. In addition, *in vivo* biomechanical environmental forces provide important stimuli that affect the formation of extracellular matrix and direct the biomechanical properties of the developing neotissue. The key steps in this process include [60]:

a) Cell proliferation and migration,
b) ECM production and organization,
c) Scaffold degradation, and
d) Tissue remodeling.

The mechanical and biological signals underlying neotissue formation remains an area of focused research. A crucial problem still to be overcome in the pediatric population is the lack of growth and remodeling potential of the grafts currently used. Multiple cell sources and seeding and culturing mechanisms have been attempted, but optimal solutions remain to be elucidated [61].

3. Tissue Engineered Vascular Grafts

The field of congenital cardiovascular tissue engineering that has advanced furthest to date is the tissue engineered vascular graft (TEVG). These conduits are used as cavo-pulmonary conduits during the final stage of the Fontan procedure (**Figure 1-2**). The goal of these conduits is the formation of a vessel that is made of native tissue that can heal, remodel, and grow as the child ages, in contrast to the currently-used conduits with no growth potential.

The first human TEVG implantations were performed in 1999 in Tokyo. The grafts used in this study were made of a woven layer of either poly-glycolic acid or poly-lactic acid with a porous inner and outer layer of poly-caprolactone/lactide. Scaffolds were seeded with patient-derived cells, the first patient receiving a graft seeded with saphenous vein cells, while the next three patients' grafts were seeded with bone marrow mononuclear cells [62]. The early success of this technique provided much hope for the field of tissue engineering and led to larger clinical studies in Japan as well as the United States.

At one year after implantation in the following Japanese trial, the grafts demonstrated a 10-20% increase in cross sectional area change from baseline, demonstrating potential growth of the neovessel within patients [63]. Intermediate follow-up demonstrated no graft related mortality, however 28% of patients developed stenosis. All stenotic patients successfully underwent angioplasty [64]. Notably, early imaging was not done on these patients unless they became symptomatic [65]. In a following clinical trial in the United States, all patients received early imaging, and asymptomatic stenosis was diagnosed and treated in three of four patients, leading to a halting of the clinical trial and a return to animal-based research for more analysis [66]. Follow-up research has since suggested that the asymptomatic stenosis seen in the United States trial was likely also present in the Japanese trial but went unrecognized as imaging was not routinely performed on asymptomatic patients. A graft explanted from a patient following a non-graft related death 13 years after implantation demonstrated a neovessel indistinguishable from the adjacent pulmonary artery or superior vena cava [45].

Follow-up studies on the clinical trial patients as well as animal work demonstrated many important factors in the development of neovessels from the grafts. In fact, mathematical modeling, as well as large animal studies, demonstrated that the early stenosis that occurred in the USA TEVG clinical trial was mathematically predicted, and interestingly was predicted to self-resolve over time as the scaffold degraded, and native mechano-mediated vessel remodeling processes could take over from the inflammation-driven reaction to the implant (**Figure 1-3**) [66]. Sheep studies confirmed these findings, demonstrating the development of asymptomatic stenosis that spontaneously resolved as the scaffold degraded. Over time, the TEVG developed histological make-up similar to that seen in the native IVC.

4. Neotissue Formation and Remodeling

The process of neotissue development is poorly understood and appears to be controlled by a multitude of factors. In some ways it mimics embryonic development whereas in other ways it appears to be governed by the rules underlying tissue repair. In fact, it is likely a unique process governed by its own set of laws. The type of cells that are implanted and their interaction with the surrounding environment determine the type of tissue that ultimately develops from the cell-scaffold complex [56].

The wide range of synthetic and natural materials used to fabricate TEHVs has led to a plethora of studies into the effects of the physical properties of the materials on neotissue formation [67]. Interestingly, recent findings suggest that microstructure morphology differences can have a profound effect on the *in vivo* response, in some cases being a stronger factor than the material used [68]. Utilization of a smaller fiber size was shown to reduce activation of contacting blood products [68]. Studies evaluating the effect of surface topography on platelet activation have found that a micropatterned rough surface is far less thrombogenic than a smooth surface [69]. Electrospun PTFE demonstrated more smooth muscle cell growth and fewer adhered platelets than a flat PTFE surface [70]. In a rat aortic graft model, aligned fibers showed significantly higher patency and less thrombus formation than a graft with a smooth topography, despite similar cellular adhesion rates to both graft types [71].

Pore size has been shown to affect cell migration, with pore sizes larger than the cells encouraging migration through the scaffold, and pore sizes significantly smaller than the cells promoting cells to adhere to the surface of the graft [72]. Degradation rate is also a critical variable to consider in the development of a tissue engineered construct; a scaffold that degrades too quickly will lead to early mechanical failure, while a scaffold that degrades too slowly may lead to stiffening and inadequate neotissue formation [67]. The mismatch of the mechanical properties between an implanted graft and the surrounding vasculature has been implicated in a number of studies as a risk factor for poor outcomes [73]. Interestingly, the adjacent vasculature has also been shown to undergo significant remodeling following graft implantation, becoming stiffer and less compliant to more closely match the properties of the graft [57, 74].

Seeded bone-marrow derived cells in TEVGs have been shown to decrease the development of neointimal hyperplasia, and were originally added under the presumption of them acting via a stem cell-like mechanism. However, after implantation seeded cells were notably seen to be lost quite rapidly from the graft after seeding, suggesting a paracrine mechanism of action rather than a function as a stem cell [75]. Recent studies of TEVGs in murine and ovine models have demonstrated that seeded mononuclear cells stimulate a robust infiltration of host macrophages during early time points [76]. Additional evidence suggests that circulating host bone marrow-derived cells are active in the acute inflammatory phase but do not represent a source of mature neotissue. Rather, macrophages appear to initiate an inflammatory cascade to drive vascular remodeling and neotissue ingrowth from the surrounding native vessel [77]. Macrophages were found to be critical to neotissue formation, with a lack of macrophages leading to a loss of neotissue formation, and an overabundance macrophages leading to higher levels of stenosis [77, 78]. These results suggest that a careful balance of the immune system is vital for optimal neovessel formation.

Targeted single photon emission computed tomography (SPECT/CT) imaging of MMP activity in TEVGs in sheep demonstrated changes in the inflammatory state of the neovessel over time as the scaffold degrades [79]. During the early phase after implantation, the graft exhibits a growing inflammatory response, as more inflammatory cells, and eventually smooth muscle cells, endothelial cells, and fibroblasts inhabit the graft. As the graft degrades, the inflammatory stimulus subsides, leaving primarily the non-inflammatory, more native vascular cell populations. In addition, this study found that bone marrow mononuclear cell seeding, often used in tissue engineering applications, had a beneficial effect at reducing early inflammation associated with neotissue overgrowth in the early phase of neotissue development.

Mathematical modeling of small animal experiments with similar implant materials demonstrated that the remodeling process is driven by two main processes: the inflammation-driven response to the implanted foreign material, and the mechano-mediated remodeling of the resulting neovessel [80]. The balance of these two factors changes dynamically over time as the stiff inflammatory graft material degrades, shifting mechanical stress and strain onto the newly infiltrating smooth muscle cells and newly deposited matrix.

5. Topics Explored in This book

As shown above, TEVGs are a promising tool for surgical treatment of congenital heart disease, but the mechanisms guiding their remodeling after implantation remain enigmatic. Historically there has been an empiric nature of design changes in tissue engineering approaches, where devices are modified on whims and experiments contain only a handful of animals. This creates difficulty in synthesizing results and creating external validity of studies, due to the interplay of mechanical and biological factors varied across studies. In order to develop a next generation of tissue engineering solutions with improved performance in both the short and long time scales, a more rational design approach must be implemented. To this end, this book seeks to individually examine several of the mechanisms at play guiding neovessel formation and remodeling, namely: mechanical properties of implanted scaffolds, biologic properties of the recipient, and the effects of long term implantation on neotissue formation and remodeling. To examine the scaffold mechanical properties as a factor in neotissue formation, we used a single breed, age, and sex of mouse in an abdominal aortic interposition model, and utilized braiding techniques to create scaffolds with identical polymeric make-up with varying mechanical properties. An aortic model was used as the mechanical stimuli in the aorta is much more dynamic and of a higher degree than that in the venous system, allowing for better visualization of any emerging effects. To evaluate the effects of biology, we next focused on the differences between male and female mice using a venous interposition model, to lessen the effect of mechanical forces. Furthermore, tamoxifen was examined as a factor in both male and female mice due to its estrogen-modulating capabilities. Finally, to better evaluate the effects of long term implantation in a more clinically-relevant model, venous interposition grafts were examined in a growing juvenile lamb model.

6. Figures

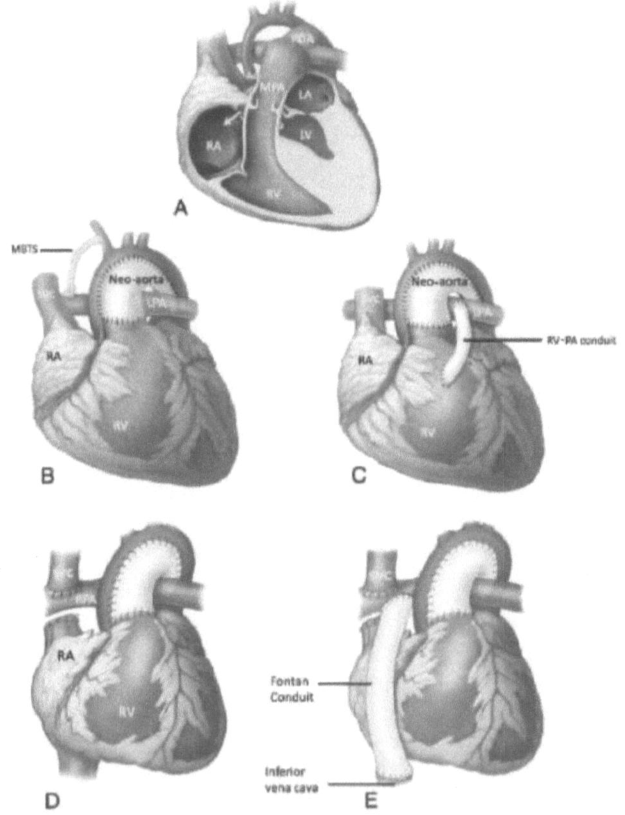

Figure 1-1 The anatomy of hypoplastic left heart syndrome with underdeveloped left ventricle (LV).

The arrow indicates the atrial septum defect. B. Stage 1 palliation using a modified Blalock-Taussig shunt (MBTS). C. Stage 1 palliation using a right ventricle (RV)–to–

pulmonary artery (PA) conduit (Sano modification). D. Stage 2 palliation using the bidirectional Glenn shunt. It is a direct anastomosis of the superior vena cava (SVC) to the right PA (RPA). E. Stage 3 palliation. The extracardiac Fontan uses a tube graft to connect the inferior vena cava to the central PA. Ao=aorta, LA=left atrium, LPA=left pulmonary artery, MPA=main pulmonary artery, PDA=patent ductus arteriosus, RA=right atrium. Reproduced from [81].

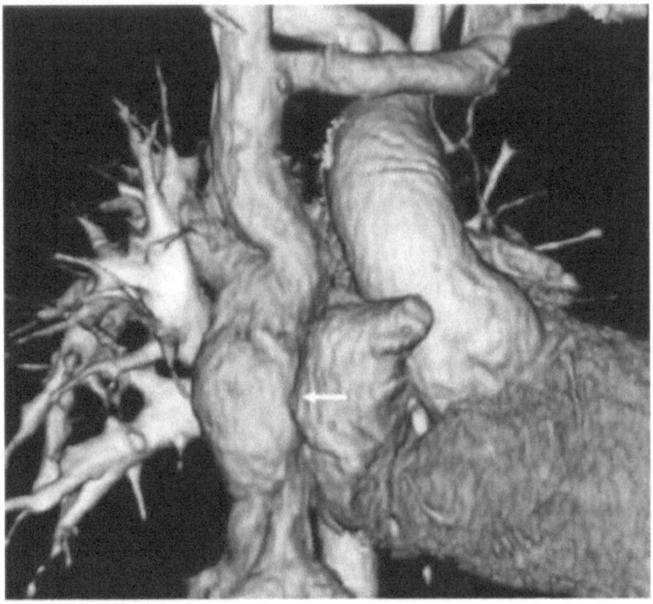

Figure 1-2 Tissue Engineered Vascular graft

Three-dimensional CT angiography of the tissue-engineered vascular graft (arrow) used as a Fontan conduit in a clinical patient. Reproduced from [64].

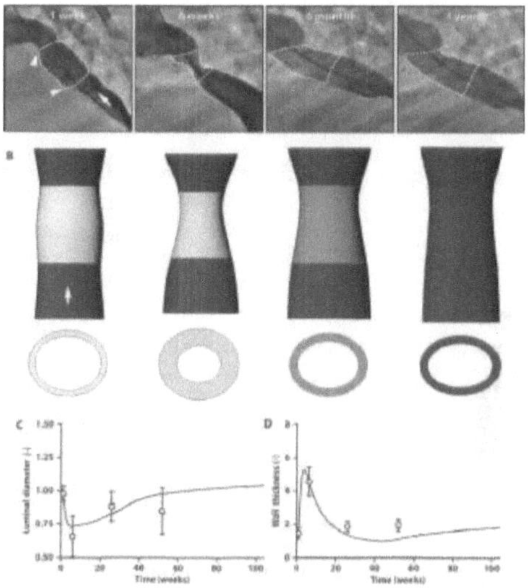

Figure 1-3 TEVG stenosis spontaneously reverses in an ovine model.

(A) Serial angiographic images of a representative ovine TEVG 1 week, 6 weeks, 6 months, and 1 year after implantation. Anastomoses are identified with white arrowheads, and the TEVG is identified by a white dotted outline. White arrow indicates direction of blood flow. (B) Image reconstructions of serial IVUS and angiographic measurements of luminal area, wall thickness, and length of the TEVG, confirming the development of stenosis at 6 weeks but spontaneous resolution by 6 months after implantation. White arrow indicates direction of blood flow. When based on lamb data, the model simulations (solid lines) for the midgraft (C) luminal diameter and (D) wall thickness fit well with the hydraulic diameters calculated from the IVUS measurements (symbols) over the 1-year study. Ovine IVUS measurements are represented as means ± SD (n = 22 at 1 week, n = 22 at 6 weeks, n = 20 at 6 months, n = 15 at 1 year). Reproduced from [66].

Chapter 2. Effects of Braiding Parameters on Tissue Engineered Vascular Graft Development

1. Introduction

There is a pressing clinical need for improved vascular conduits, particularly small caliber arterial grafts. Coronary and peripheral bypass procedures commonly utilize autologous vascular grafts, which have demonstrated 10-year patencies of 60-90% depending on the procedure and the vessel used [82-84]. However, about one-third of patients lack suitable autologous vessels due to pre-existing conditions or previous operations [85, 86]. Tissue engineered vascular grafts (TEVGs) offer a unique solution, allowing fabrication of off-the-shelf vascular conduits that can develop into functional blood vessels within the body [87, 88]. While several TEVGs have been translated to the clinic, performance has been mixed and design improvements have largely been based on empiricism rather than rational design, thus hindering clinical development [88, 89]. An ideal TEVG needs to be readily available, easily implantable, biocompatible, resistant to thrombosis, stenosis and dilation, as well as capable of developing into a living functional neovessel [90]. These factors depend heavily on both the scaffold materials used and the manufacturing method.

Poly(glycerol sebacate) (PGS), also known as "biorubber," is the first biodegradable polymer designed specifically for fabricating TEVGs [91]. It is biocompatible, nonthrombogenic, and highly elastic, which is ideal for an artificial arterial conduit [91]. It also demonstrates a sufficient degradation profile to allow adequate time for neotissue formation without remaining so long as to cause a longstanding foreign body reaction; it undergoes complete degradation *in vivo* within approximately 6 weeks [92]. Despite the broad range of potential applications and scientific interest towards PGS, its difficulties in manufacturing and handling have hindered its entry to the clinic [93]. By contrast, poly(glycolic acid) (PGA) is a long-used biomaterial, particularly in TEVGs, which degrades within 12 weeks *in vivo*, though with loss of mechanical integrity occurring between 4 and 8 weeks [80, 94, 95]. Novel scaffolds can easily be envisioned that combine the advantages of each of these important biomaterials, but the question is, how best to design new scaffolds?

Computational modeling has shown promise for accelerating the optimization process of vascular grafts by determining potential mechanisms of neotissue formation and effects of altering scaffold parameters [96, 97]. Recent models informed by experimental data have suggested that *in vivo* neovessel formation is an inflammation-driven, mechano-mediated process [80]. Therefore, altering the design of the scaffold provides a two-fold means for optimizing *in vivo* performance. More specifically, the chemical, mechanical, and morphometric properties of a scaffold can be changed to modulate the degree of induced inflammation, with particularly critical properties including polymer chemistry, fiber size and alignment, pore size, porosity, and degradation rate [98]. The evolving mechanical properties are especially important as they can dictate the degree of stress shielding of cells within the developing neotissue, thus affecting mechanobiologically mediated extracellular matrix production, remodeling, and degradation [74]. Importantly, factors that define the inflammatory status and mechanical properties of a scaffold are strongly coupled, making selection of individual parameters more challenging and the creation of an optimized design elusive. Successful neovessel formation requires neotissue development to balance scaffold degradation. Lack of coordination between these processes can lead to pathologic remodeling or graft failure.

While computational modeling offers a potential way to predict optimal scaffold parameters, improvements in fabrication methods with a high degree of control and replication will similarly be necessary to realize optimal designs [96, 99]. Textile manufacturing offers a well-established method for producing scaffolds from a broad array of biodegradable polymers that can be fabricated with a wide range of mechanical properties. Textile manufacturing allows certain degrees of decoupling of the chemical and mechanical properties of the scaffold, enabling a wide range of mechanical properties using the same polymer yarn. Braiding, in particular, offers a tunable platform for fabricating scaffolds, allowing precise selection of complex anisotropic mechanical profiles [90]. Increasing the braid angle relative to the axial direction increases the circumferential stiffness of the scaffold, while decreasing the axial stiffness. Picks per square inch (PPSI) and number of ends together determine the void space within the braid with increases of either parameter decreasing void space therefore increasing the bulk stiffness of the graft. Braiding also allows tissue-level mechanical properties to be decoupled from those at the cellular level by utilizing identical polymer fibers woven in different arrangements. In this study, we investigate braiding as a method for producing PGA scaffolds having different immunogenic and mechanical properties. These scaffolds were manufactured with and without PGS coating. Scaffolds were evaluated in a Beige mouse model and implanted in the infrarenal abdominal aorta (IAA). By selecting scaffold designs that represent current bounds of what is manufacturable/testable, we demonstrate that, for the same polymer chemistry, differences in initial physical/mechanical properties can alter neotissue formation as well as graft performance. Such data will prove critical in informing the next computational models for accelerating design.

2. Results

2.1 Scaffold Fabrication

Parameters of each graft design are listed in **Table 2-1**. Braiding parameters included braiding angle, number of ends, and PPSI. Braiding angle is defined as the angle between the clockwise and counterclockwise fiber bundles, and the number of ends is the total number of fiber bundles used to create the braid. PPSI refers to the number of cross overs seen in a given surface area of the braid. 1x1 and 2x2 refer to the braiding style used, where a 1x1 braid has 1 clockwise bundle crossing over a single counterclockwise bundle, and a 2x2 has 2 clockwise bundles crossing over 2 counterclockwise bundles. **Figure 2-1** provides an overview with representative scanning electron microscope (SEM) images of each scaffold design, gross images of a TEVG at implantation and explantation, and a timeline of measurements and testing.

2.2 Survival

The mechanism of failure differed across the different scaffold designs (**Table 2-2**). Within the 1x1 braiding designs, scaffolds with low PPSI, which results in looser braids, demonstrated higher rates of early death from surgical bleeding and early ruptures, often within the first week. The Design 1 cohorts, which have a denser braid (i.e., high PPSI), had only one bleeding death in each group, and no early ruptures. However, the uncoated Design 1 group had two mice die from a later rupture, at 28- and 46-days post-implantation. Due to the different incidences of graft failure modes, 12-week survival ranged from 29% to 93% depending on design, with the coated dense braid of Design 1 performing the best. There were no deaths in any group between 7 and 26 days (**Figure 2-2**). At explant, all surviving animals demonstrated patent lumens with no evidence of thrombosis.

Designs 4 and 5 were manufactured using a 2x2 braiding pattern, and 10 mice per cohort were initially implanted. Surgical deaths from anastomotic bleeding ranged from 1-3 animals per group (**Table 2-2**). The Design 4 cohort did not experience early rupture, but four coated and three uncoated grafts experienced aneurysmal dilation and rupture between days 27 and 38. With the Design 5 cohort, 7 of 9 animals died due to bleeding through the graft within the first week. Due to the high mortality in this group, the uncoated version was not implanted. The high failure rates, and differential modes of failure, suggested a need for a tighter braid to prevent early bleeding and provide more structural support during degradation. As such, only the 1x1 braided designs were used for the remainder of the studies.

2.3 Serial Ultrasound & Blood Pressure Monitoring

Ultrasound analysis detected a rapid increase in diameter between weeks 4 and 8, with diameters remaining steady beyond 8 weeks (**Figure 2-3**). Design 2 grafts demonstrated earlier dilation than the other designs, possibly due to its looser, smaller angle braid. Representative 3D models for all graft designs can be seen in **Figure 2-4**. All grafts demonstrated low compliance in comparison to baseline measurements of the native aorta. Compliance remained low over time, even following degradation of the scaffold (**Figure 2-5**). Proximal and distal anastomotic changes were minimal (**Figure 2-6**). Blood pressure monitoring, performed on the ultrasound analysis cohorts, demonstrated no differences in blood pressure across groups or over time (**Figure 2-7**).

2.4 MMP Activity and Inflammation

General matrix metalloproteinase (MMP) analysis, using an MMP-activatable fluorescent probe, demonstrated low signal in the grafts at 12 weeks (**Figure 2-8a**), with results similar across groups (**Figure 2-8b**). Inflammation was assessed by cluster of differentiation 68 (CD68) antibody staining (**Figure 2-8c**), a pan-macrophage marker. The effect of coating was found to be significant ($p = 0.0098$) on fractional area of CD68 staining, while direct statistical comparisons between groups were not significant. With the exception of the Design 3 coated and uncoated cohorts, all groups had significantly higher expression of CD68 compared to that the native aorta (**Figure 2-8d**).

2.5 Biaxial Mechanical Testing

Measured unloaded outer diameter and wall thickness were greater for all grafts than the age-matched native IAA. All varied significantly except for the diameter of coated grafts of Design 1 and 3 and the thickness of Design 3 coated grafts (**Figure 2-9b-c**). Both Design 2 uncoated and coated cohorts had significantly different *in vivo* axial stretch compared with the native aorta ($p = 0.03$, $p = 0.04$, respectively) (**Figure 2-9d**). All grafts had a significantly different measure of distending elastic energy (energy associated with loading the vessel from 10 to 140mmHg, at *in vivo* axial stretch) ($p = 0.03$ for D1 coated, $p = 0.04$ for the other groups) (**Figure 2-9e**). The grafts also had significantly different measures of distensibility compared to the native aorta ($p < 0.001$ for all) (**Figure 2-9f**). While significant differences in mechanical and morphological properties were observed between all graft designs and the native IAA, no significant differences were observed among the different grafts. Finally, despite the relatively large increase in compliance compared to the scaffolds at implantation, all the explants remained much stiffer structurally than the age-matched native IAA.

2.6 Structural Histology Quantification

Figure 2-10a shows representative images of sections stained using techniques for Hart's, Picro-Sirius Red (viewed under polarized light), and calponin. Quantification of the positive area fraction of Hart's elastin (**Figure 2-10b**) showed differential effects of scaffold design on elastin density, which were significant ($p < 0.001$) while the effect of coating was not ($p = 0.294$). Specifically, significant differences in elastin density were seen between Design 2 (low braiding angle) and the other two designs (both high braiding angles) for both uncoated and coated cohorts. All groups, except Design 2 uncoated and coated cohorts, had significantly lower elastin densities compared to the native aorta. Measurements of the overall thickness of elastic laminae provided further insight into elastin deposition [100]. The effect of graft design was also significant ($p < 0.001$), and like elastin density, Design 2 uncoated and coated cohorts were significantly thicker compared to the other designs (**Figure 2-10c**). Interestingly, Design 2 had a thicker elastic lamina compared to the native aorta, with significant differences seen between the Design 2 uncoated cohort and the native aorta ($p = 0.0031$).

The effect of graft design on Picro-Sirius Red staining for collagen fibers was marked. Design 1 had a significantly greater collagen density compared to Design 2 for both uncoated ($p < 0.001$) and coated ($p < 0.001$) cohorts (**Figure 2-10d**). Design 2 samples also had a significantly lower collagen density in comparison to the native aorta for both uncoated ($p < 0.001$) and coated ($p = 0.003$) cohorts. The effect of scaffold design was significant regarding mature smooth muscle cell density ($p = 0.0022$) as reflected by the fractional area of calponin staining but showed no significant differences between any groups (**Figure 2-10e**). This also includes comparison between the TEVGs and the native aorta. All quantified measurements were normalized to total areas to account for differences in size between grafts and native aortas samples. Non-normalized data can be found in the supplement (**Figure 2-11**). These data show similar differences between graft designs. Finally, only one sample, a Design 2 uncoated graft, was positive for calcification, seen with both von Kossa and Alizarin red staining (**Figure 2-12**).

2.7 Statistical Relations

By logistic regression, the 2x2 scaffolds associated with a higher rate of overall mortality ($p > 0.001$). Increasing the braiding density of the scaffold by increasing the PPSI decreased mortality, whereas increasing the braiding angle resulted in higher mortality. Despite seeing an increase in mortality in some PGS coated groups, coating was not found to statistically affect survival beyond normal surgical variation. Multiple linear regression on the explanted 1x1 scaffolds (Designs 1, 2 and 3) evaluated the effect of scaffold braiding parameters on neovessel development. Increasing the PPSI correlated with decreased elastin and increased collagen density. Increasing the braiding angle towards a more circumferential braid correlated with a decrease in elastin, an increase in collagen, and a decrease in both calponin and CD68 positive cells. Increasing the angle also correlated with a decreased distensibility of the vessel by mechanical testing at explant. The addition of the PGS coating correlated with an increase in collagen and a decrease in inflammatory CD68 positive cells. Statistical details of these regressions can be found in **Table 2-3**.

Regression analysis of the quantitative histology of the explanted vessels further demonstrated interesting relationships (**Table 2-4**). Elastin and collagen were inversely related, as expected because area fractions, by definition, must sum to 1 and elastin and collagen are the primary constituents of the extracellular matrix. Elastin and calponin positive cells, elastin and CD68 positive cells, and calponin and CD68 positive cells correlated positively with each other. Comparing histology to mechanical testing data from the same animals demonstrated that there was no correlation between calponin or CD68 positive cells and distensibility. In contrast, elastin correlated positively with distensibility

(p = 0.029) while collagen showed a near inverse correlation with distensibility (p = 0.054).

3. Discussion

We used 12-week implantations to evaluate specific bounds of the manufacturable parameter space for braided PGA scaffolds with and without a PGS coating. The differential temporal progressions of neovessel development and modes of graft failure (e.g., anastomotic bleeding, early or late rupture) remind us of the importance of evaluating degradable TEVGs across their full degradation time course as different mechanisms are likely operative at different times. Indeed, previous computational simulations of short-term implants reinforced the importance of following the long-term performance of tissue engineered vascular grafts [99, 101].

In a study using electrospun scaffolds of poly-ε-caprolactone-co-L-lactic acid fibers (PCLA), all arterial grafts experienced sudden dilation and rupture at 14 weeks due to the sudden loss of mechanical strength of the scaffolds and inadequate tissue formation [99]. A study utilizing an electrospun PGS scaffold reinforced with an external poly(ε-caprolactone) (PCL) sheath only showed vascular architecture after 12 months *in vivo* while still exhibiting high levels of inflammation due to the slowly degrading PCL sheath and small pore sizes for the inner PGS layer. Similar PGS-PCL scaffolds showed peri-operative mortality of over 30% thought to be due to defects in the outer sheath and the increased coagulability of wild-type mice [101, 102]. In both studies of bilayered PGS-PCL scaffolds, mechanical testing after 12 weeks of implantation revealed low distensibilities in comparison to that of native vessels, as in the present study. Modification of the microstructural design of the PGS-PCL scaffolds in these studies required changes to the entire electrospinning protocol and were met with a number of challenges, including wrinkling and luminal occlusion due to swelling. The use of textile manufacturing methods in this study allowed finer control over graft parameters without major modifications to the fabrication process; use of faster degrading polymers, PGA and PGS, showed the capacity for swifter neovessel development.

The *in vivo* imaging methods used in this study included advanced volumetric ultrasound strategies that allowed us to better assess *in vivo* graft performance. For example, we collected 3D ultrasound images at multiple timepoints, through which we determined graft diameters and thicknesses. While diameter can be determined from standard 2D images, the 3D datasets provide a more holistic view of graft development, as has been shown previously in murine aneurysm studies [103-105]. Of particular interest, we noted a thickened wall in Design 1 at week 4, which thinned by week 6 and remained stable for the rest of the study. Despite the thickened wall at week 4, we did not observe any narrowing of the lumen consistent with stenosis. These results were confirmed with histology at week 4, which showed little tissue formation on the luminal surface of the scaffolds but substantial collagen deposition surrounding the braided scaffolds (**Figure 2-13**). We believe this initial adventitial collagen deposition is responsible for the increase in thickness seen on ultrasound at 4 weeks. This suggests that this graft design may be undergoing rapid remodeling between weeks 4 and 6. We also observed an increase in diameter at the proximal and distal ends of some grafts, resulting in a barbell shape. While not observed in all animals, this may suggest faster graft degradation and neotissue formation at the anastomoses relative to the middle of the graft, consistent with infiltration of native vascular cells from the adjacent vessels [77]. Finally, using M-mode ultrasound, we calculated low strain within the graft while the native IAA proximal and distal to the graft remained highly pulsatile, indicating a relatively consistent strain gradient across the anastomoses. Given that this strain gradient likely changes throughout the remodeling process, future work with 4D ultrasound (3D+time) could enable noninvasive assessment of strain along the vessel [105, 106]. Overall, the advanced 3D ultrasound metrics included in this study gave us greater insight into graft remodeling compared to standard imaging approaches.

Beige mutant mice were selected for their relative platelet storage pool deficiency compared to wild-type mice [107]. Previous studies by our laboratory showed benefits of using Beige mice to prevent early thrombosis in the small diameter vascular grafts evaluated in mice [108-110]. Higher thrombosis rates are expected in murine grafts compared to large animal grafts, as smaller arterial diameter greatly increases platelet shear stress [111, 112]. Others have also shown that wild-type mice have hyperactive platelet responses compared to humans and larger animals such as rats [113, 114]. The use of a mouse model with platelet storage pool deficiency thus allows examination of molecular and cellular mechanisms that drive neotissue formation without the confounding high thrombosis rates that would be seen in a wild-type mouse.

The explanted neovessels demonstrated high levels of elastin deposition. This result is notable as the vast majority of TEVGs, whether made from decellularized matrix or synthetic polymers, have difficulty in triggering elastin production [115]. Individual elastin fibers in the native aorta appear wavier than fibers seen in the neovessels due to the dilation of the grafts. The Design 2 cohorts had a similar elastin density to that of the native aorta. These cohorts also experienced steady dilation compared to the rapid dilation in other cohorts. Increasing (cyclic) wall tension associated with dilation could be one reason for increased elastin density in these groups [116, 117]. However, these cohorts had thicker elastic laminae with thinner fibers in comparison to native vessels, which may suggest that the elastin fibers are immature or not organized fully. It is uncertain if they would develop further, though continued elastin deposition from 3 to 6 months has been observed [102]. The elastin in the grafts appears to be more organized than what has been seen in previous studies looking at the same time point in PGS-PCL grafts [101, 102, 118]. Nevertheless, the elastin in each of these graft designs is not serving its functional capacity due to the low energy storage capacity observed in these stiff constructs. Smooth muscle cells also appear circular compared to the elongated cells of the native aorta which could indicate these cells are in a synthetic, noncontractile state, indicating ongoing extracellular matrix remodeling [119]. Notably, calponin-positive cells were only present within the neotissue closest to the lumen. Previous studies have also observed contractile cells within the neointima of tissue engineered vessels [120].

Statistical regression analysis comparing the implanted scaffold parameters to the explanted neovessel characteristics demonstrated that the PGS coating decreased inflammation and increased collagen accumulation. The lower inflammation and macrophage density seen at explant (12 weeks), in comparison to other polymer-based vascular grafts at similar time [75, 100, 101], likely reflected the near complete degradation of polymer by 12 weeks. PGA fibers appear birefringent under polarized light [66], and the fibers were seen in 4-week explants but not at 12-weeks, suggesting complete degradation of the polymer by 12 weeks (**Figure 2-13**). While macrophages and inflammation are essential for neotissue formation, macrophage overabundance or prolonged inflammatory response associates with worse outcomes for tissue engineered vessels [75]. Slow degrading polymers, expectedly, associate with longer lasting inflammation and more foreign body giant cell formation [121]. Overall these findings suggest that the differences in scaffold designs affected the balance of immuno-driven and mechano-mediated matrix production in development of the neovessels. This aligns with our previous study that used computational modeling to demonstrate how you can change inflammation and alter neotissue in a predictable manner by altering scaffold morphometry [98]. The low incidence of calcification seen in this study is also likely related to the shorter polymer degradation times, as nondegradable conduits highly susceptible to calcification after long implantation [122]. In a previous study in rats, adding a PGS coating to a PGA arterial scaffold decreased the incidence of calcification and improved the inflammatory response seen with a shift in macrophage polarization [100]. While we have not specifically examined the molecular mechanism PGS may have on inflammation, for similar biodegradable scaffolds we have demonstrated this is a TGF-β mediated process [123].

Our study further demonstrated that increasing the braiding angle towards the circumferential direction decreased distensibility at 12 weeks. Although one expects decreased distensibility with preferential circumferential polymer fiber alignment early on, this finding after degradation of polymer reinforces the thought that polymer orientation influences cell alignment, and thus, neotissue alignment. Notwithstanding the deposited elastin and the positive correlation between elastin content and distensibility, the *in vivo* axial stretch and energy stored elastically upon pressurization were both considerably lower in the grafts than in native IAAs, consistent with the elastin not being fully functional, the presence of excessive, stiff collagen, or both. The non-native organization of the elastic laminae and the trend toward a negative correlation between collagen content and distensibility suggests that both are likely. The ability to store energy elastically is critical to the function of conduit vessels such as the aorta and remains an unmet need. While the grafts evaluated in this study did not reach the compliance of the native aorta, they developed to levels similar to those seen in aneurysmal murine arteries [124-126]. This may be due to the initial stiffness of the implanted scaffolds, thus a more compliant scaffold may have facilitated mechanical properties that better match the native vessel. Recall, also, that the more compliant scaffolds evaluated in this study, the 2x2 braided designs, were still significantly less compliant than a native vessel and had a high failure rate due to the lack of structural integrity, both initially and over the course of degradation. Thus, finding the appropriate balance between initial stiffness and strength remains a significant challenge.

Overall, statistical regression analysis of the relations between scaffold characteristics and neovessel outcomes highlights the complexity and importance of rational design in tissue engineering. While many tissue engineering design improvements are made empirically to improve a specific parameter, such as amount of collagen deposited or reduced inflammation, we can see from the statistical regressions (**Table 2-3 & 2-4**) that many of these parameters, such as survival, collagen deposition, and inflammation, are intertwined in both their relation to scaffold design parameters and their relations to each other. For example, increasing the density of a scaffold by increasing the PPSI served to improve survival, but it also decreased elastin production. Similarly, decreasing the braiding angle towards the axial direction improved distensibility and survival, but led to early dilation as seen by ultrasound. In addition, changing of braiding parameters can have unintended consequences, such as loosening of the overall braiding structure, which can lead to a higher rate of bleed through as was seen in Designs 4 and 5 with the 2x2 braiding pattern. Careful balancing of the relative importance of multiple desired parameters will be necessary to determine a proposed ideal scaffold with optimized performance in both the short and long-term after implantation in a patient [96].

4. Conclusion

In this work, braided small-diameter arterial grafts of PGA with and without PGS coating were manufactured at the edges of the braidable parameter space and evaluated for failure mode and performance within a murine IAA implantation model. Braiding parameters, and the resulting physical properties of the scaffolds, had a substantial effect on the success and failure mode (i.e., bleeding, early rupture, late rupture) *in vivo*. Braiding parameters and PGS coating also affected the histological make-up of the resulting neovessels. Detailed ultrasound analysis allowed longitudinal *in vivo* evaluation of morphometric properties and explant biaxial testing allowed functional consequences of immunohistological findings to be contextualized. Statistical findings from this work will aid in the development of mathematical models to predict the outcomes of new scaffolds.

5. Experimental Section

5.1 Graft Fabrication

6.1.1 Scaffold Braiding

Scaffolds were braided on a mandrel with an outer diameter of 0.66 mm by a 48-carrier braider (Steeger USA; Inman, SC) using 45 denier, 20 filament PGA yarn (Riverpoint Medical; Portland, OR). All scaffold designs were fabricated using a 1-ply design and a 0.3 mm tension spring setting and were scoured in 99% isopropyl alcohol at ambient temperature for 15 minutes. The 1x1 and 2x2 designs were heat set for 1.5 hours at 180°C and 1 hour at 130°C, respectively.

6.1.2 Poly(glycerol sebacate) Coating and Curing

PGS coating solutions were made by mixing 23 g of molten PGS (Regenerez® Secant Group, LLC; Telford, PA) with 77 g of ethyl acetate (Sigma 319902) in an 8 oz polypropylene jar (Uline; Pleasant Prairie, WI) using a stir bar and stir plate set to 500 RPM for 2 hours. The homogenous PGS coating solution was transferred to a 50 mL graduated cylinder and positioned under the arm of the Single Vessel dip coater (KSV NIMA; Gothenburg, Sweden). Approximately 20 cm lengths of each design were cut from their mandrels and fastened to the dip coating arm. Two rounds of dip coating in the PGS polymer solution were performed for the coated graft cohorts, with a 15-minute drying period between rounds. Grafts were cured in a vacuum oven (JEIO TECH OV-12) at 120°C and 10 torr for 18 hours. All grafts were sterilized by gamma irradiation (18-29 kGy dosage).

5.2 Scanning Electron Microscopy

Scaffold samples were prepped for scanning electron microscopy by mounting with carbon tape. Samples were then imaged under low vacuum using JEOL JSM 1060LA Scanning Electron Microscope under 10kV, a spot size of 60%, and a working distance of 10 mm.

5.3 Implantation

All animal experiments were approved by the Nationwide Children's Hospital and Purdue University Institutional Animal Care and Use Committee and all animals received humane care in compliance with the National Institutes of Health (NIH) *Guide for the Care and Use of Laboratory Animals* (NIH, Bethesda, MD, USA). Beige mice (C57BL/6J-Lyst$^{bg\text{-}J}$/J; The Jackson Laboratory, Bar Harbor, ME, USA) between 8-12 weeks of age, were used for surgery (n=10-15 per group). Scaffolds 3 mm long were implanted as IAA interposition grafts using standard microsurgical technique facilitated by an operating microscope with zoom magnification [127]. Briefly, a midline laparotomy incision was made from below the xyphoid to the suprapubic region, and a self-retaining retractor inserted. The intestines were wrapped in sterile saline-moistened gauze and retracted. The aorta was separated from the inferior vena cava and vascular control was obtained with microvascular clamps. The IAA was transected. Scaffolds were implanted, anastomosed proximally and distally with 10-0 polypropylene running suture. The skin was then closed in two layers by using a 6-0 black polyamide monofilament suture, and animals were moved to a recovery cage with a warming pad until becoming fully ambulatory.

5.4 Ultrasound Analysis

Mice (n=2-4 per group based on surgical survival) were imaged using high frequency ultrasound (Vevo3100; FUJIFILM VisualSonics Inc., Toronto, ON, Canada) before surgery, as well as 1, 2, 4, 6, 8, 10, and 12 weeks post-implantation. During imaging, mice were anesthetized with 1-3% isoflurane and placed supine on a heated stage. Hair was removed from the abdominal region using chemical depilatory cream (Nair, Church & Dwight, Ewing, NJ). A 22-55 MHz frequency linear transducer was used to acquire long- and short-axis brightness (B-) mode, motion (M-) mode, and ECG-gated Kilohertz Visualization images of the IAA at locations proximal, mid, and distal to the graft (MS550D, FUJIFILM VisualSonics). Additionally, a linear step motor was used to collect sequential 2D short-axis images to create 3D datasets. The luminal and adventitial boundaries were segmented manually from the volumetric image data using the open source code SimVascular to create 3D representations of the grafts. The segmentations were then imported into MATLAB (MathWorks, Natick, MA) to calculate the effective diameter at each z-slice location along the graft. In addition, thickness was determined from 2D short-axis images at the mid-graft location (VevoLAB, FUJIFILM VisualSonics). We calculated circumferential Green-Lagrange strain using the M-mode images by measuring systolic and diastolic diameters in triplicate.

5.5 Blood Pressure Measurements

Blood pressure was measured at baseline before implantation, and again at 4, 8, and 12 weeks post-implantation using a CODA 2 Channel Standard Blood Pressure System (Kent

Scientific, Torrington, CT). For each mouse (n=2-4 per group), at least 10 replicate measurements of systolic, diastolic, and mean arterial pressure were averaged per timepoint.

5.6 MMP Activity

To measure general MMP activity, 100μL of MMPSense™ 680 (PerkinElmer, Waltham, MA) was injected via tail vein approximately 24 hours prior to euthanasia. After euthanasia, the graft and aorta were placed under near infrared light (625 nm excitation; 700 nm emission) to obtain fluorescent images from both the dorsal and ventral sides (4000mm Digital Imaging Station, Kodak). Using a custom MATLAB script, the intensity ratio for each image was calculated as the ratio of signal intensity in the graft relative to that of the healthy aorta [124]. Dorsal and ventral regions were averaged to give a single value per mouse (n=2-4 per group).

5.7 Biaxial Mechanical Testing

The entire IAA, including the graft, was explanted and stored in Hanks Balanced Salt Solution at 4°C until mechanical testing, performed within 72 hours of harvest. These composite vessels (n=2-4 per group), were cannulated and secured to paired glass pipettes using 6-0 suture [101]. The mounted vessels were placed in a custom computer-controlled biaxial testing system in Hanks Balanced Salt Solution and the unloaded dimensions (length and outer diameter) were recorded at 10 mmHg [128]. The preconditioning protocol is similar to that for the native IAA and included equilibration at 90 mmHg with low intraluminal flow at *in vivo* stretch for 15 mins, followed by pressurization from 10-140 mmHg for 4 cycles [129]. The unloaded dimensions of the vessels were measured again after preconditioning and the *in vivo* stretch of the composite vessels were estimated by identifying the axial stretch at which axial force was nearly constant in response to a change in pressure. The protocol for pressure-distension tests similarly involved cyclic pressurization of the vessels from 10-140 mmHg at a constant vessel-specific *in vivo* stretch, while the protocol for axial force-extension tests involved loading from 0 to 25 mN axial force at a fixed pressure. Distensibility calculations are based on external diameter measurements. Force and pressure were measured using standard transducers; axial stretch was controlled using a sub-micron resolution stepper motor, and diameter was tracked using a video-camera and custom software. Native IAAs of similar length from 20-week-old Beige mice were used for the control group.

5.8 Histology & Immunohistochemistry

Following either MMP-Sense or mechanical testing, grafts were segmented into transverse sections and samples were fixed in 10% formalin and paraffin-embedded. Sections 4 μm thick were stained using standard techniques. Hart's elastin stain was used to evaluate elastin density and thickness, Picro-Sirius Red was used to assess collagen density, and von Kossa and Alizarin Red were used to detect calcification, if any (n=4-13 per group, based on surgical survival).

For immunohistochemistry, tissue sections were deparaffinized, rehydrated, and blocked for endogenous peroxidase activity and non-specific protein adsorption prior to staining. Primary antibodies and associated concentrations were calponin (Abcam 203047, 1:100) and CD68 (Abcam 125212, 1:2000). Slides were stained with appropriate secondary antibodies at a concentration of 1:1500 followed by incubation in streptavidin horseradish peroxidase (Vector). Color development was performed with 3,3-diaminobenzidine (Vector) and tissue was counterstained with Gill's hematoxylin. Photomicrographs were acquired with a Zeiss AxioObserver.Z1 inverted microscope with a 20x objective and captured with a Zeiss Axiocam 105 (color) digital camera.

Image analysis was performed using ImageJ (National Institute of Health, MD, USA) [130, 131]. Images from two different segments of each graft were analyzed and averaged. Quantification evaluated elastin layer thickness, elastin density, collagen density, calponin positive area fraction, and CD68 positive area fraction. Area measurements were obtained by pixel-specific thresholding based on specific values of hue, saturation, and brightness as well as size. The reported densities or area fractions correspond to the number of positively defined pixels over the total number of pixels in the vessel region.

5.9 Statistical Analysis

Results are presented as mean values ± standard deviations. Ultrasound data were analyzed using a repeated measures two-way ANOVA (main effects of graft and time) with a post-hoc Dunnett's test. For other data, statistical significance among groups was determined using ANOVA with post-hoc Dunnett's or Sidak's tests for multiple comparisons based the standard deviation of the data. We considered $p \leq 0.05$ to be statistically significant. Statistical analyses were performed with GraphPad Prism 8.0 (GraphPad Software, CA, USA).

Regressions were performed using STATA statistical software. Multiple linear regressions were performed for each histological analysis as well as for explanted vessel distensibility.

Independent variables defining the scaffold designs were PPSI, Braiding Angle, and Presence of PGS coating (as a Boolean variable). Again, a $p \leq 0.05$ was used as a level of significance for each regression term. Logistic regression was used for each of the 5 implanted designs to determine the effect of scaffold parameters on survival. Independent variables were type of braid (2x2 vs 1x1), PPSI, braiding angle, and presence of PGS coating. Number of ends and mass/inch were initially included as independent variables but were determined to be covariate and subsequently removed from the analysis.

6. Conflicts of Interest

C.K.B. is an inventor on patent/patent applications [2015252805 (Australia), 2016565483 (Japan), 855,370, 9,446,175, 9,782,522, 10,300,082, 61/987,910, 62/266,309, 62/309,285, 62/209,990, 62/936,225] submitted by Yale University and/or Nationwide Children's Hospital that cover methods of improving the design, manufacturing, or performance of tissue-engineered vascular grafts. C.K.B. is a founder of Lyst Therapeutics.

9. Figures and Tables

Table 2-1 Manufacturing Parameters of Braided TEVGs

Design	**Braid Pattern**	**Number of Ends**	**Picks per Square Inch [PPSI]**	**Braiding Angle**	**Mass per Inch [mg]**
1	1 x 1	24	19110	83	4.1
2	1 x 1	24	7350	38	3.2
3	1 x 1	12	7350	107	2.6

4	2 x 2	24	29400	107	5.1
5	2 x 2	32	13230	38	4.3

Summary of braiding parameters utilized to create the braided TEVGs in this study.

Table 2-2 Summary of Implants.

Design	**Coated [Y/N]**	**Number Implanted**	**Bleeding Deaths**	**Early Ruptures [≤1 Week]**	**Late Ruptures [>3 Weeks]**	**Survival at 12 Weeks**
1	Y	14	1	0	0	93%
	N	14	1	0	2	79%
2	Y	14	3	3	0	57%
	N	15	3	2	0	67%
3	Y	14	6	4	0	29%
	N	15	5	3	0	47%
4*	Y	10	1	0	4	50%
	N	10	3	0	3	40%
5*	Y	10	1	7	0	20%

N	0	-	-	-	-

Summary of the total number of implants performed and associated morbidity and mortality. Base scaffolds were PGA; coating was with PGS. * Implants of 2x2 designs were limited due to mortality events associated with the looseness of the braid.

Table 2-3 Regression Outcomes.

	2X2	PPSI	Angle	PGS
Survival	- (<0.001)	+ (<0.001)	- (0.04)	ns
Elastin	N/A	- (0.003)	- (<0.001)	ns
Collagen	N/A	+ (<0.001)	+ (0.002)	+ (0.006)
Calponin	N/A	ns	- (0.004)	ns
CD68	N/A	ns	ns	- (0.007)
Distensibility	N/A	ns	- (0.027)	ns

Each regression is plotted as a specific row, with independent variables in separate columns. (+) and (-) denote a relation being significant with a direct or inverse relation, with the associated p-value in parentheses. ns denotes Not Significant (p>0.05).

Table 2-4 Histological Comparisons.

	Collagen	Elastin	Calponin
Elastin	- (<0.001)		
Calponin	ns	+ (<0.001)	
CD68	ns	+ (0.011)	+ (0.009)

Direct regressions of row and column histological findings for all explanted vessels. (+) and (-) denote a relation being significant with a direct or inverse relation, with the associated p-value in parentheses. ns denotes Not Significant (p>0.05). Duplicate and blank columns removed for clarity.

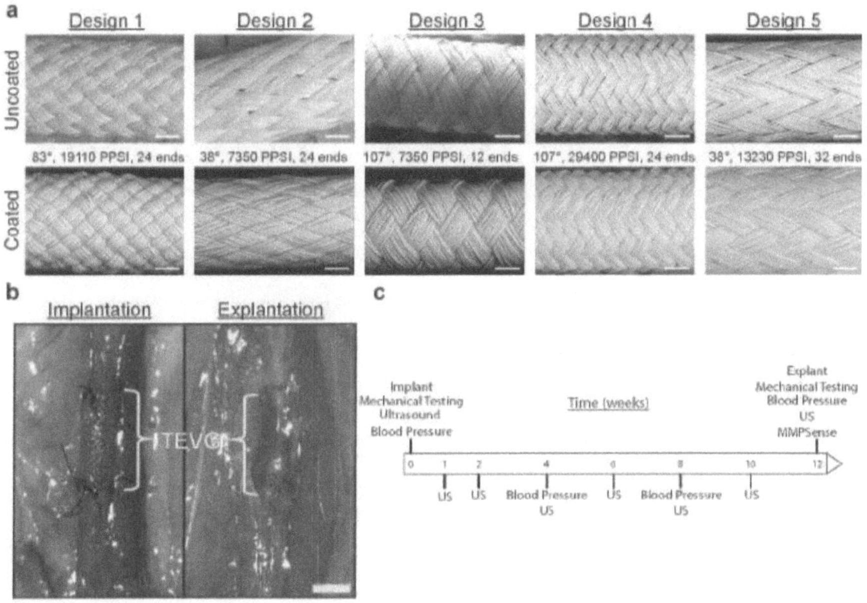

Figure 2-1 Experimental Overview

a) Representative SEM images of the five graft designs with the listed braiding parameters showing both PGS coated and uncoated cohorts. White scale bar = 200 μm. b) Images of the braided TEVG upon implantation in the infrarenal aorta and 12 weeks later upon explantation. Yellow scale bar = 2 mm. c) Experimental timeline.

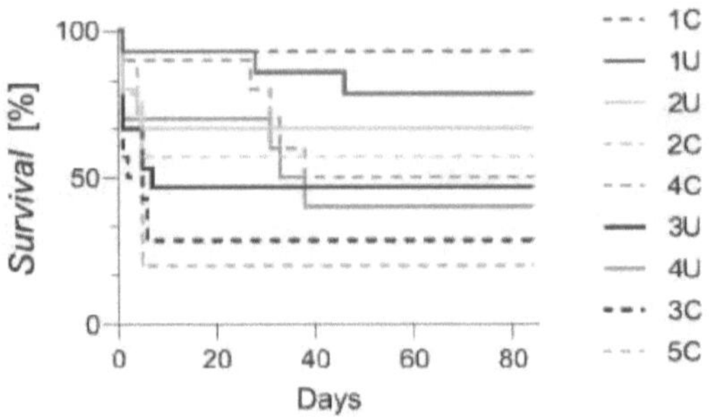

Figure 2-2 Survival Curve

Survival varied over time. Three time points showed the greatest drops in survival, all due to different modes of graft failure. The initial deaths (< 0 days) were found to be due to anastomotic bleeding. Other early deaths (1-7 days) were due to grafts dilating slightly, which created an opening between braids and resulted in internal bleeding. Later deaths (>26 days) were caused by rapid dilation of the graft upon degradation, which resulted in graft rupture and internal bleeding.

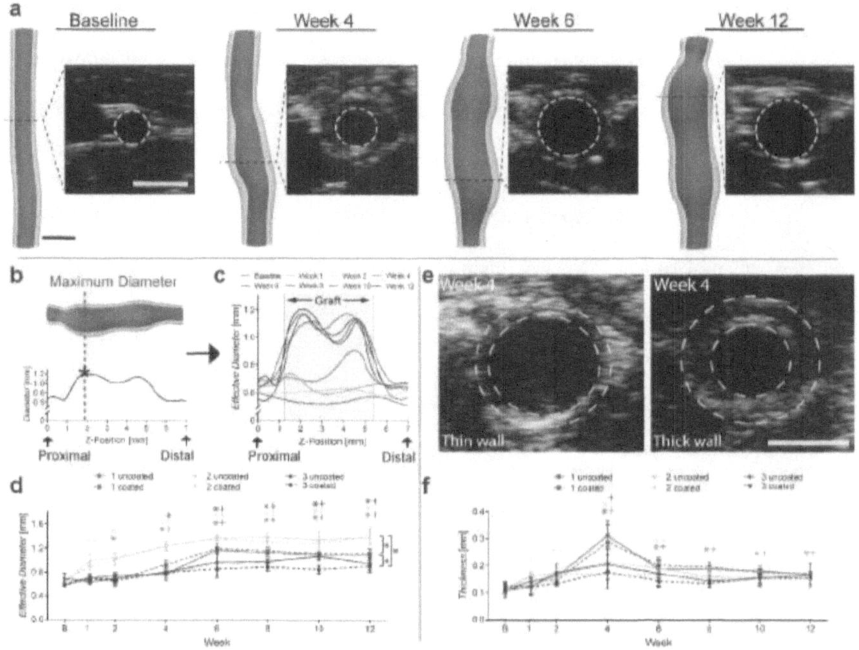

Figure 2-3 Ultrasound Analysis of Diameter and Thickness

a) Representative segmentations were developed from 3D ultrasound images and highlight graft remodeling over time. This particular progression was for a mouse with a Design 1 coated graft. b) Segmentations were then used to calculate effective lumen diameter at every z-slice of the graft, and c) for each time point. d) Maximum lumen diameter varied per group, with Design 2 showing an early increase, while Design 1 had an abrupt increase between weeks 4 and 6. Design 3 had the smallest diameter at the end of study. e) In addition, representative ultrasound images show the difference between thin-walled

(Design 2) and thick-walled (Design 1) grafts, as was quantified in (f). Dashed lines demarcate the luminal and abluminal boundaries of the graft and are shown for illustrative purposes. Actual measurements were performed in VevoLAB and SimVascular. An '*' refers to uncoated and a '+' refers to coated, with the color indicating the appropriate group ($p < 0.05$). All comparisons are relative to baseline. n = 2-4 per group. Data were compared using two-way ANOVA (main effects of graft and time) with a post-hoc Dunnett's test. Scale bars = 1 mm.

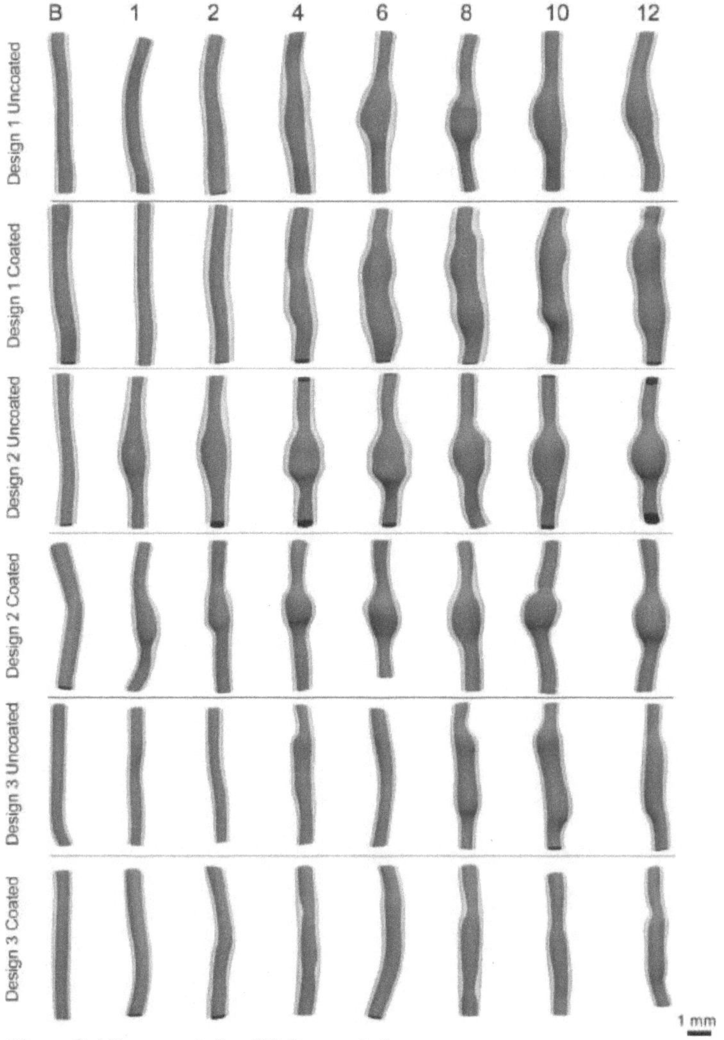

Figure 2-4 Representative 3D Segmentations

Volumetric representations from each vessel show the remodeling process of each graft type over 12 weeks. Diameter and strain were measured from the ultrasound images at locations proximal and distal to the graft, as well as at the location of the maximum diameter within the graft. An '*' refers to uncoated and a '+' refers to coated, with the color indicating the appropriate group ($p < 0.05$). All comparisons are relative to baseline.

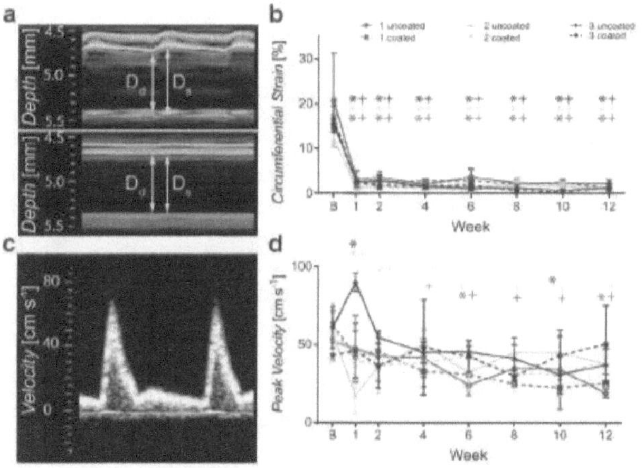

Figure 2-5 Ultrasound Analysis of Strain and Velocity

a) *In vivo* cyclic circumferential Green-Lagrange strain was determined from M-mode images. b) All groups had an immediate reduction in strain following implantation of the scaffold that remained low throughout the study. c) Peak velocity was quantified from pulsed-wave Doppler ultrasound and d) showed some small changes, though highly variable. Representative images were taken from a Design 1 coated (for a) and uncoated (for c) graft, but similar results were observed for all graft types. An '*' refers to uncoated and a '+' refers to coated, with the color indicating the particular design ($p < 0.05$). All comparisons are relative to baseline. n = 2-4 per group. Comparisons were made with two-way ANOVA (main effects of graft and time) with a post-hoc Dunnett's test.

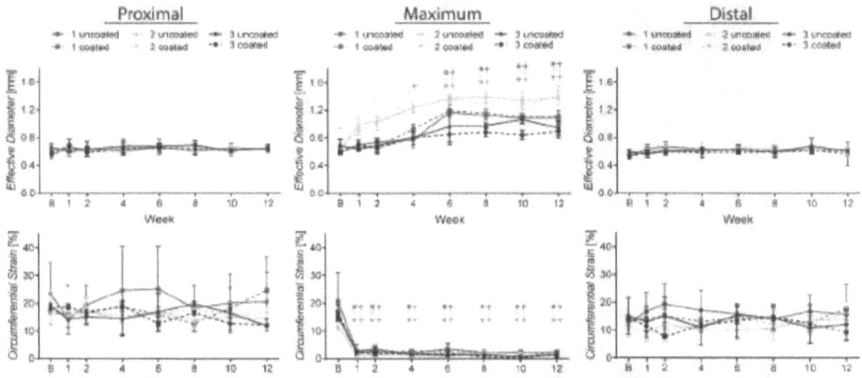

Figure 2-6 Ultrasound-Based Diameters and Strains

Full diameter and strain measurements from ultrasound analysis for Designs 1, 2, and 3. Actual measurements were performed in VevoLAB and SimVascular. An '*' refers to uncoated and a '+' refers to coated, with the color indicating the appropriate group ($p < 0.05$). All comparisons are relative to baseline. n = 2-4 per group. Data were compared using two-way ANOVA (main effects of graft and time) with a post-hoc Dunnett's test.

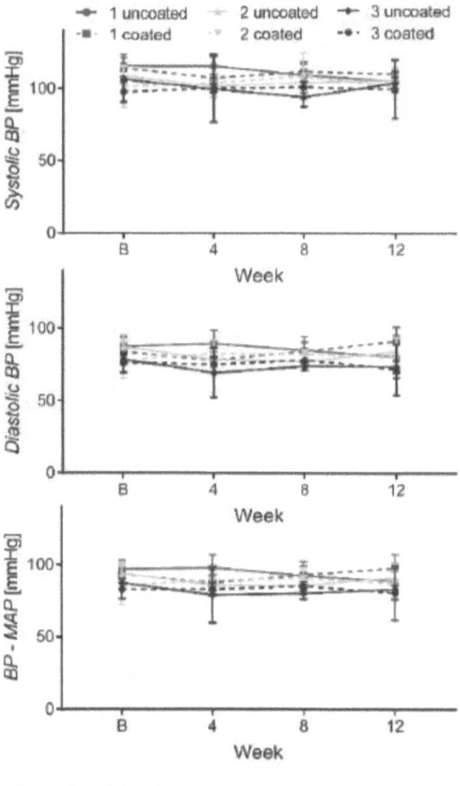

Figure 2-7 Blood Pressure Measurements

Systolic, diastolic, and mean arterial blood pressure were unaffected by graft implantation, as demonstrated by the lack of significant differences among groups or compared to baseline.

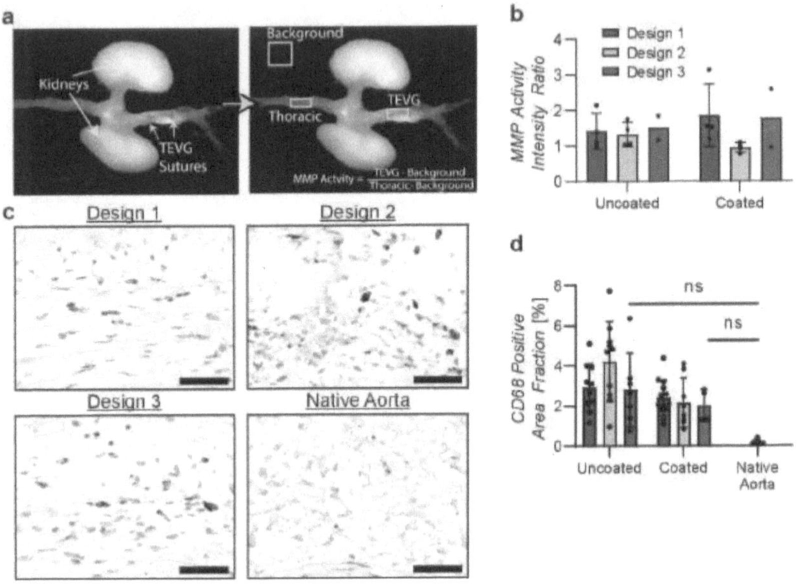

Figure 2-8 MMP Activity and Inflammation

a) Using near-infrared images of the explanted aorta/graft complex, MMP activity was calculated as the ratio of average TEVG intensity to thoracic intensity, after removing the effect of the background. These representative images were taken from a Design 1 uncoated mouse. b) Results indicated that MMP activity was not different between designs or coatings. n = 2-4 per group. Comparisons were made with ANOVA. c) Immunohistochemical staining using an antibody specific for CD68, a pan-macrophage marker. Representative images taken using a 63x objective. Scale bar = 40 μm. d) Results showed no significant differences between graft designs. Designs 1 and 2 both had significantly higher CD68 expression compared to the native aorta for both uncoated (D1;

$p < 0.001$, D2; $p = 0.002$) and coated (D1; $p < 0.001$, D2; $p = 0.03$) grafts while Design 3 did not for uncoated ($p = 0.08$) and coated ($p = 0.11$). n=4-13 per group, based on survival. Comparisons were made with ANOVA with a post-hoc Dunnett's test.

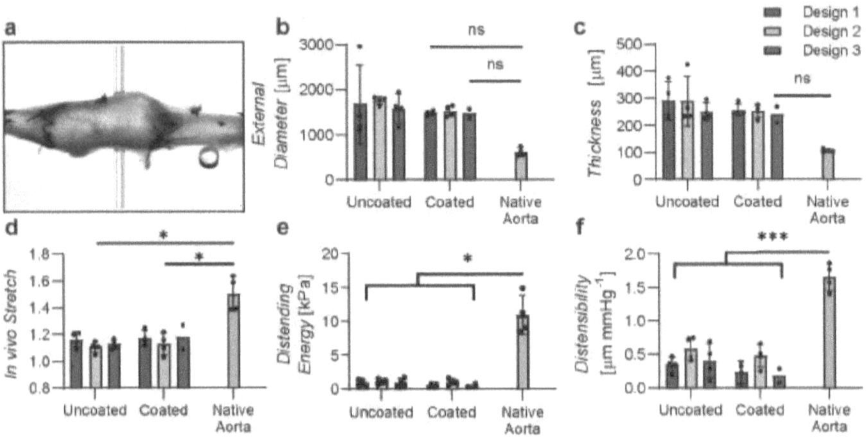

Figure 2-9 Biaxial Mechanical Properties

a) External diameter tracking of a representative explanted TEVG during biaxial mechanical testing upon explantation at 12 weeks. This representative image was taken from a Design 1 coated mouse. b-f) Summary of mechanical properties of graft designs (n = 4 for all groups except Design 3 coated which had n = 2). For external diameter, coated Design 1 and 3 were the only groups found to not be significantly different than the native aorta ($p = 0.06$, $p = 0.22$ respectively). Similarly, the coated Design 3 group was the only one found not significantly thicker than the native aorta ($p = 0.1$). Design 2 uncoated and coated cohorts had significantly different values of *in vivo* stretch compared to the native aorta ($p = 0.03$, $p = 0.04$ respectively). All groups had significantly different measures of distending energy (that due to distension alone) and distensibility compared to the native aorta. While significant differences in mechanical and morphological properties were observed between all graft designs and the native IAA, no significant differences were observed across graft designs. Comparisons were made with ANOVA with a post-hoc Sidak's or Dunnett's test depending on standard deviation. (* < 0.05, ** <0.01, *** <0.001)

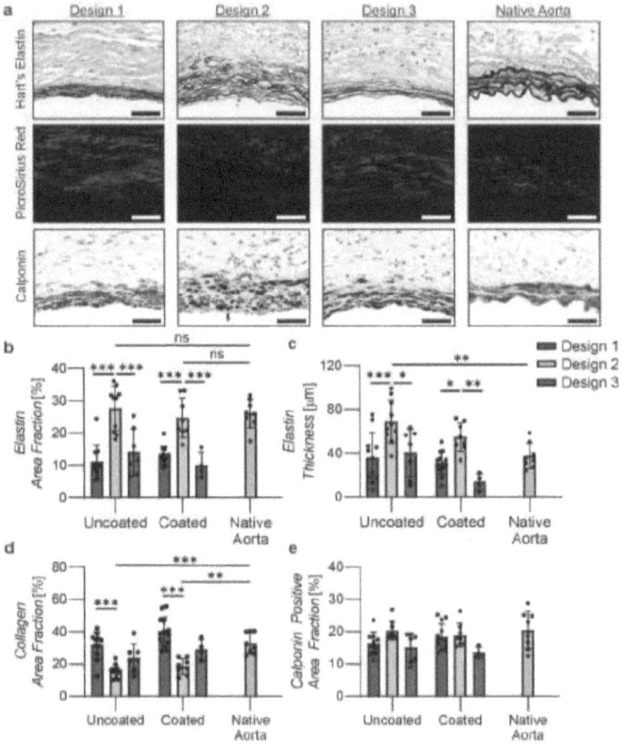

Figure 2-10 Histological Analysis

Representative histological and immunohistological images of all graft designs followed by images of a native aorta. Stains include Hart's for elastin, Picro-Sirius Red for collagen, and calponin for smooth muscle cells. Images were taken using a 63x objective. Scale bars = 40 µm. b-c) evaluation of Hart's elastin showed differences in both elastin density and elastic lamina thickness between Design 2 and Designs 1 and 3 for coated and uncoated cohorts. Design 2 coated and uncoated cohorts were the only groups that did not have significantly decreased elastin density compared to the native aorta. Design 2 uncoated was the only group that had a significantly thicker band of elastin compared to the native aorta. d) Design 1 coated and uncoated cohorts had significantly higher densities of collagen when compared to the Design 2 cohorts. The Design 2 cohorts both had significantly lower collagen densities compared to the native aorta. e) No differences in smooth muscle positive area fraction were observed between any group or to the native aorta. n=4-13 per group. Comparisons were made with ANOVA with a post-hoc Sidak's test. (* < 0.05, ** <0.01, *** <0.001)

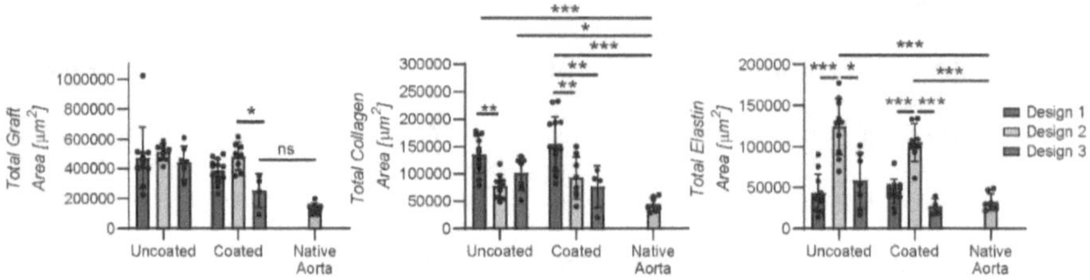

Figure 2-11 Total Area Histological Analysis

Graphs show total area measurements from histological samples. The first graph is the total tissue area of the vessels stained with Picro-Sirius Red and imaged with brightfield microscopy. Design 2 and 3 coated were the only Designs to differ significantly (p =0.03). Design 3 coated was also the only group to not significantly vary from the native aorta (p = 0.78). All other grafts had significantly greater tissue area ($p < 0.001$ for all groups). The second graph shows the collagen area measurements from vessels stained with Picro-Sirius Red and imaged with polarized light. Design 1 grafts contained significantly greater amounts of collagen compared to Design 2 for both uncoated ($p = 0.006$) and coated ($p = 0.004$) cohorts. Similar results were seen between Design 1 and 3 but only for the coated cohort ($p = 0.04$). Design 1 grafts, both uncoated and coated, as well as Design 3 uncoated grafts had significantly greater amounts of collagen compared to the native samples ($p < 0.001$, $p < 0.001$, $p = 0.04$ respectively). The last graph shows the total elastin area measurements from the Hart's elastin stain. Design 2 uncoated and coated groups had greater amounts of elastin compared to the other designs and the native aorta ($p = 0.02$ between D2 and D3 coated, $p < 0.001$ for all other groups). n=4-13 per group. Comparisons were made with ANOVA with a post-hoc Sidak's or Dunnett's test. (* < 0.05, ** <0.01, *** <0.001)

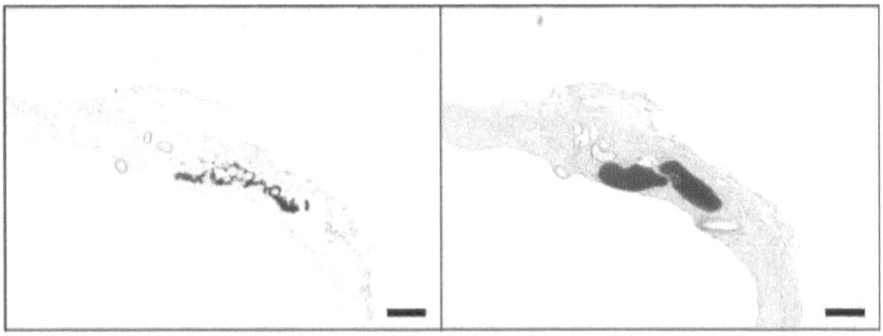

Figure 2-12 Calcification

Representative image of calcification from von Kossa and Alizarin Red staining. The graft is from the Design 2 uncoated cohorts. Images were taken using a 20x objective. Scale bar = 100 μm.

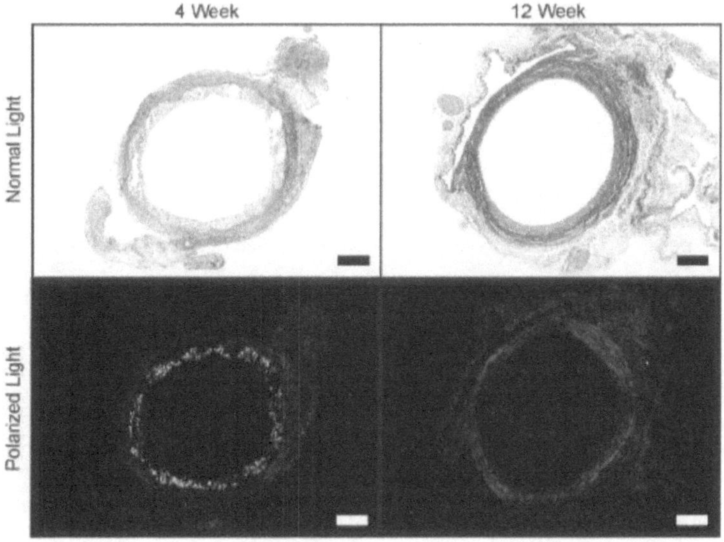

Figure 2-13 Fiber Degradation

Representative images of grafts at 4 and 12 weeks stained with Picro-Sirius Red and imaged with normal and polarized light. These are Design 1 coated grafts. At 4 weeks, PGA fibers show up clearly under polarized light due to their birefringence. At 12 weeks there is no indication of fibers remaining upon examination with polarized light. It is possible that PGA polymer still exists in the wall but there does not appear to be any large fibers providing mechanical support. Images were taken using a 20x objective. Scale bar = 200 μm.

Chapter 3. Tamoxifen Confounds Cardiovascular Tissue Engineering

1. Background

Tissue engineered vascular grafts (TEVGs) represent a promising development in vascular surgery [65]. These polymer-based conduits which degrade over time and are replaced by native tissue, resulting in the formation of a functional blood vessel made from the patient's own cells. However, the precise cellular mechanisms underlying the development of TEVG neotissue remain to be elucidated [65]. Genetic mouse models are a powerful tool to study these processes because of their ability to manipulate cellular pathways both temporally, through the use of tamoxifen- and diphtheria-induced models, and spatially, through the use of cell-specific models [132-134].

Tamoxifen, a selective estrogen receptor modulator, has wide-spread use as a small molecule effector for inducible knock-out models [135]. This system works by fusing a Cre-recombinase to an estrogen receptor (Cre^{ERT2}) that resides in the cytosol until activated. Activated CRE^{ERT2} then translocates to the nucleus, where Cre induces recombination and subsequent knock-out of any gene modified with flanking Lox-P sites [136].

Direct tamoxifen binding can weakly activate estrogen receptors, however its metabolites, formed through CYP2D6 enzymes within the liver, are much more biologically active [137]. Recently, several studies have identified that tamoxifen may have a confounding impact on mouse models. A single low dose of tamoxifen in wild type male mice was shown to have long term effects on testes and endocrine function [138]. Tamoxifen also dampened the inflammatory response and accelerated skin wound healing in ovarectomized females [139]. In the liver, tamoxifen attenuated hepatotoxicity, increased levels of antioxidants, and increased the presence of immune cells [140]. While utilizing tamoxifen-driven Cre^{ERT2} mice in a unilateral uretal obstruction model, tamoxifen was found to confound experimental results [141]. Specifically, tamoxifen attenuated fibrosis in female kidneys, but not male kidneys, even if tamoxifen injections were halted 14 days prior to the renal injury. In contrast, for neurologic models tamoxifen treatment via oral or IP administration did not affect behavior, cell proliferation, cell survival, or dendritic arborization in male or female mice [142].

It is not surprising that tamoxifen may have predictable off-target effects. Estrogen signaling is highly interconnected with many cellular signaling pathways, including proliferation, invasiveness, and apoptosis, which have effects far beyond the target tumor in cancer therapy [143]. Selective estrogen receptor modulators such as tamoxifen are also known to have variable tissue-specific effects, acting as an antagonist in breast tissue, but as a partial agonist in bone, uterine, and heart tissue [144]. In humans, tamoxifen is primarily used in estrogen receptor positive breast cancer treatment for which it has a potent antitumor effect, but also has off-target effects including a pro-tumorigenic effect on endometrial tissue, predisposing to thrombotic events such as deep vein thrombosis [145]. Tamoxifen also leads to decreases in blood cholesterol, triglyceride levels, leukocyte levels, and platelet levels, and an increase in the incidence of radiotherapy-induced lung fibrosis [145-147].

Estrogen has an important role in wound healing and fibrosis, inhibiting macrophages and downregulating pro-inflammatory phenotypes [148]. As an estrogen modulator, it is therefore unsurprising that tamoxifen has shown effects in many fibrosis models in both humans and animals. Tamoxifen treatment in humans decreases the formation of hypertrophic scars *in vivo*, and *in vitro* decreases human fibroblast contraction of collagen matrices [149, 150]. In pigs, tamoxifen has also been shown to limit fibrosis in a common bile duct anastomosis model [151]. Tamoxifen treatment in rats decreased fibrosis in pulmonary and nephrosclerosis models [152, 153]. In a mouse model or tubulointerstitial fibrosis, tamoxifen decreased fibroblast proliferation, extracellular matrix deposition, and inflammation [154]. Effects on fibrosis are presumably through mediation of TGF-β signaling, a cytokine known to play an important role in fibrosis, scar formation, and wound healing, as well as neotissue formation in tissue engineering [155-157].

To date, no studies have examined the effect of tamoxifen in the context of tissue engineering. In addition, while tamoxifen is widely used in laboratory conditions for conditional knock-out models, it is often assumed to be inert in the systems being studied; a potentially hazardous assumption considering the number of studies examining its effects directly. In order to evaluate the potential effect of sex on neotissue formation as well as confounding effects of tamoxifen, we implanted tissue engineered vascular grafts in both sexes of mice with and without tamoxifen treatment and evaluated the resulting neotissue.

2. Results

2.1 Mouse Survival and Surgical Outcomes

In order to determine the sex-specific effects of tamoxifen on TEVGs, 8-10 weeks old male and female mice were administered a tamoxifen chow or control chow diet one week before TEVG implantation as an infrarenal inferior vena cava (IVC) interposition graft (**Figure 1A-D**). Mice were kept on this diet throughout the evaluation period until sacrifice at two weeks post implantation. Two weeks was chosen as the study end date as we have previously reported this as a key time point for determining long term TEVG outcomes in mice [75].

Male mice, as expected, were larger than their age-matched female counterparts at each time point (**Figure 1E**). On the date of surgery, one week after beginning treatment, tamoxifen chow led to a significant decrease in weight relative to control animals in both males and females (males 23.5±1.6 vs 19.4±3.2 g, $p<0.01$; females 18.6±1.0 vs 13.2±1.9 g, $p<0.001$), a known phenomenon due to food avoidance[158]. By the 2-week post-surgery explant date, the body weight of female mice had recovered and were no longer different from untreated female mice (20.0±1.0 vs 19.5±1.4 g, $p=0.22$). Interestingly, male mice on tamoxifen chow treatment remained at a lower weight than their controls at the time of sacrifice (24.7±2.1 vs 21.2±1.4 g, $p<0.001$).

Tamoxifen treatment had an effect on surgical survival in both male and female mice (**Figure 1F**). While untreated animals had 100% surgical survival, both male and female mice treated with tamoxifen experienced deaths occurring during the surgical recovery period (first 24 hours post-implantation), although this difference was not significant for either sex individually (**Figure 1G**). Interestingly, male mice on tamoxifen experienced deaths in the days prior to surgery, presumably related to their observed weight loss. Tamoxifen treatment had an effect on increasing the TEVG occlusion rate in female mice (from 25% to 62%, $p<0.05$), however, male mice were unaffected with equal occlusion rates in both groups (25% vs 13%, $p=0.67$) (**Figure 1H**).

Due to the significant weight loss seen in the tamoxifen-treated mice, an additional cohort of female mice was implanted with daily tamoxifen treatment delivered by intraperitoneal (IP) injection. Female mice administered with tamoxifen by IP injection did not experience weight loss and surgical survival matched untreated mice (100%), but the occlusion rate was not different from the tamoxifen chow group (65%, $p<0.05$ vs female untreated controls). These observations suggest that weight loss was due to food aversion to the tamoxifen chow, surgical deaths were weight loss related, and occlusion was due to tamoxifen treatment and not due to weight loss, respectively.

2.2 Neotissue Formation

Hemotoxylin & eosin (H&E) and Picro-Sirius Red (PSR) staining of the resulting neotissue demonstrated differences in cellularity and extra cellular matrix (ECM) production, respectively, in TEVGs between untreated males and untreated females (**Figure 2A-C**). TEVGs implanted into untreated males had decreased cellularity compared to untreated females (4206±623 female vs 3611±633 male cells/mm^2, $p<0.01$) (**Figure 2D**), and markedly decreased collagen deposition (4.6±1.4 vs 1.6±0.4 area percent, $p<0.001$) (**Figure 2E**). Collagen maturity was also decreased in untreated male mice compared to untreated females (46.0±9.0 female vs 36.7±11.8 male percent mature, $p<0.05$) (**Figure 2F**).

Tamoxifen had several effects on female mice. Cellularity was decreased in female mice on tamoxifen compared to female controls (4206±623 control vs 3146±568 chow vs 2436±330 IP cells/mm^2, $p<0.001$ for IP and chow compared to control) (**Figure 2D**). Tamoxifen decreased tissue area in females compared to untreated females (61.1±5.4 control vs 51.1±11.9 chow vs 45.3±5.2 IP area percent, $p<0.01$ control vs chow, $p<0.001$ control vs IP) (**Figure 2G**). Collagen area was decreased in females on tamoxifen chow compared to untreated females (4.6±1.4 control vs 2.2±0.8 chow area percent, $p<0.001$) (**Figure 2E**). Female mice on IP tamoxifen showed decreased collagen maturity (46.0±9.0 control vs 31.0±4.9 IP percent mature, $p<0.05$) (**Figure 2F**).

Due to known effects on wound healing and fibrosis, TGF-β1 and TGF-β3 gene expression were measured by reverse transcription quantitative real time polymerase chain reaction (RT-qPCR). TGF-β1 (**Figure 2H**) and TGF-β3 (**Figure2I**) expression were not significantly different between males and females, although TGF-β1 expression was lower in IP tamoxifen treated females compared to untreated females (1.00±0.09 control vs 0.82±0.04 IP relative gene expression, $p<0.05$). The ratio of TGF-β1 to TGF-β3, however, was lower in untreated males compared to untreated females (5.48±0.75 female vs 3.16±0.82 male TGF-β1 / TGF-β3 ratio, $p<0.01$) (**Figure 2J**). While there was a trend towards decreasing the TGF-β1/β3 ratio with tamoxifen treatment in females and increasing in males with tamoxifen treatment, the effects were not significant.

Cellular proliferation marker Ki67 (**Figure 2K**) was higher in untreated males compared to untreated females (0.31 ± 0.05 female vs 0.44 ± 0.06 positive cell fraction, p<0.001). In addition, tamoxifen treatment decreased Ki67 expression in both sexes (females 0.31±0.05 control vs 0.26±0.06 chow vs 0.22±0.05 IP, p<0.01; males 0.44±0.06 control vs 0.39±0.05 chow, p<0.05).

2.3 Estrogen Receptor Markers

Estrogen receptor alpha (ER-α) and estrogen receptor beta (ER-β) were downregulated by tamoxifen treatment in females as measured by both immunohistochemical staining (**Figure 3A-D**) and RT-qPCR (**Figure 3E,F**). ER-α histology staining was decreased in females with tamoxifen treatment and in untreated males compared to untreated females (female 3.4±1.7control vs 1.6±0.8 chow vs 0.7±0.4 IP percent positive area, p<0.01 control vs chow, p<0.001 control vs IP; male 1.9±1.7 vs 3.1±2.2 control; p<0.05 male vs female). ER-α gene expression was reduced in females with tamoxifen (female 1.03±0.25 control vs 0.65±0.22 chow vs 0.57±0.05 IP relative gene expression, p<0.05 control vs chow, p<0.001 control vs IP). ER-β histology was only decreased in females (14±5 control vs 8±3 chow vs 7±3 IP percent positive area, p<0.001 for each vs control). ER-β gene expression was decreased in females with tamoxifen chow (1.08±0.43 control vs 0.51±0.11 chow relative gene expression, p< 0.05).

2.4 Cellular Make-Up of Neotissue

At two weeks, all explanted TEVGs demonstrated complete endothelialization of the midgraft lumen (**Figure 4A**). Within the walls of the TEVG, small vasa vasorum could also be seen by staining of endothelial cell junctions with anti-CD31 antibody (**Figure 4B**). The density of these vessels was not different between males and females, but was decreased in females with tamoxifen chow treatment compared to untreated females (225 ± 63 vs 131 ± 20 vessels/mm^2, $p<0.05$) (**Figure 4D**). Desmin, a marker of fibroblasts and immature smooth muscle cells, showed marked decrease in expression in females given IP or chow tamoxifen treatment (females 12.04±4.16 control vs 6.76±4.21 chow vs 9.22±2.08 IP area percentage, $p<0.001$ control vs chow, $p<0.05$ control vs IP) (**Figure 4C,E**). RT-qPCR for additional markers of fibrosis and smooth muscle cells, FSP-1 and αSMA, showed little to no differences between groups, with the exception of FSP-1 having decreased expression in tamoxifen IP females compared to untreated females (1.01±0.13 control vs 0.45±0.10 IP relative gene expression, $p<0.001$) (**Figure 4F,G**). Male gene expression of FSP-1 and αSMA also showed more within group variation than was observed for females.

2.5 Inflammatory Response to TEVG Implantation

CD68 was used as a pan-macrophage marker, staining both macrophages and foreign body giant cells (**Figure 5A**). While the levels of CD68 expression were similar between untreated males and females, there was a marked difference in the formation of foreign body giant cells in response to the TEVG, with males having much lower giant cell formation (65 ± 24 vs 29 ± 11 giant cells/mm^2, $p<0.05$). Tamoxifen treatments in female mice decreased levels of both macrophages (601 ± 80 control vs 447 ± 36 chow vs 502 ± 106 cells/mm^2, $p<0.001$) and giant cells (65 ± 24 control vs 39 ± 11 chow vs 43 ± 14 IP cells/mm^2, $p<0.05$) (**Figure 5B,C**).

The degradation of the TEVG biomaterial, as assessed by imaging for graft fibers under polarized light (**Figure 2B,C**) was also different between sexes (**Figure 5D**), with males RT-qPCR for inflammatory M1 (NOS2) (**Figure 5E**) and anti-inflammatory M2 (Arg1) (**Figure 5F**) macrophage markers demonstrated no significant differences between groups. In addition, the NOS2/Arg1 ratio was quite low in all groups, suggesting a heavily anti-inflammatory macrophage phenotype (**Figure 5G**). NOS2/Arg1 ratio in female mice on IP tamoxifen was decreased (0.040 ± 0.013 control vs 0.008 ± 0.004 IP, $p<0.01$). Monocyte chemoattractant protein 1 (MCP-1) gene expression was increased in both male and female mice on tamoxifen relative to controls (females 1.02 ± 0.21 control vs 1.88 ± 0.34 chow vs 1.64 ± 0.53 IP relative gene expression, $p<0.01$ control vs chow, $p<0.05$ control vs IP; males 0.67 ± 0.25 control vs 1.51 ± 0.65 relative gene expression, $p<0.05$ control vs IP) (**Figure 5H**), notable as macrophage levels were not increased in any treatment groups. MMP-9 gene expression was decreased in males relative to females (1.05 ± 0.33 females vs 0.39 ± 0.05 males relative gene expression, $p<0.05$), and decreased in females on IP tamoxifen relative to control (1.05 ± 0.33 control vs 0.31 ± 0.17 IP relative gene expression, $p<0.05$) (**Figure 5I**).

3. Discussion

Improving our understanding of the biomechanical, cellular, and molecular pathways underlying neotissue formation in TEVGs holds the key to improving their performance through rational design. A lack of effective and correlative biological implantation models hinders the translation of tissue engineering findings, as the differences in geometry, mechanics, and biological signaling between humans and research animals must be considered[159]. A history of empiric design changes and studies using a small number of animal models has made comparisons between studies difficult and further hinders a mechanistic understanding of tissue engineering paradigms [160]. Fine-tuning of mechanical and microstructural scaffold parameters can vastly alter biological outcomes [96, 102]. However, even when engineering factors affecting scaffold creation are tightly controlled, biologic factors such as sex and age can play a significant role in altering outcomes in TEVGs, demonstrating a need for careful and detailed evaluation of biological experimental models and their baseline assumptions and limitations [161, 162]. In this study, we have shown multiple effects of sex on a cardiovascular tissue engineering model, as well as sex-specific effects of tamoxifen. Sex-specific differences in untreated mice, particularly in cellularity, deposition of neotissue, development of giant cells in reaction to biomaterial implantation, and differences in rate of biomaterial degradation have strong consequences towards the development of ideal tissue engineering solutions.

Human studies have shown differences in the estrogen pathways as well as in inflammatory state between the sexes in untreated animals. Female patients are more susceptible to inflammatory and autoimmune disorders such as asthma, and higher numbers of macrophages and a stronger inflammatory response are typically seen in women [163]. Additionally, in human macrophages, ER-α and ER-β are present in males and females, and are higher in males [164]. Levels of monocytes and macrophages in blood and tissues are shown to be different across males and females, and across various mouse strains used in research [165]. Prior studies have further demonstrated that estrogen exerts different effects on males versus females. Studies in mice found that estrogen given to ovarectomized mice can reduce MCP-1 and leukocyte infiltration, suggesting that estrogen acts as a reprogramming switch for macrophages to turn from M1 to M2 by acting through ER-α [166]. The same study found that post-menopausal women have increased M1 response, with similar M2 response, shifting the M1/M2 balance [166].

Results in this study related to the inflammatory response further this understanding and go on to suggest that macrophages and monocytes of males and females respond differently to implanted biomaterials, an important consideration for evaluation of biomaterials as well as their translation to the clinic. Females create more foreign body giant cells and produce more collagen. Males, on the other hand, degrade the implanted biomaterial much more rapidly despite similar levels of macrophages. The large difference in the inflammatory response between sexes compared to similar M1/M2 ratios seen in this study may suggest that additional factors related to macrophage and monocyte function in response to biomaterials should be investigated in future studies.

In addition to sex differences in tissue regeneration and remodeling, we showed that tamoxifen treatment alters the host response to TEVGs. Tamoxifen has previously been shown to prevent endothelial cell migration and proliferation in a rat model, and while estrogen can accelerate the re-endothelialization of denudated carotid arteries, tamoxifen does not have this effect [167, 168]. This is corroborated by our findings in this work in female mice, where Ki67-labeled proliferation and CD31-labeled endothelial cell expression were decreased at two weeks in our TEVGs. Interestingly, male mice treated with tamoxifen also had a decrease in Ki67 expression.

Throughout early experiments, the significant weight loss associated with the tamoxifen chow treatment raised concern of weight loss and malnutrition being causal of the findings in this study, as opposed to effects of tamoxifen directly, as decreased cellularity and increased inflammation have been seen in these states [169, 170]. Malnutrition has been shown to interact with many important wound healing pathways, including upregulation of IL-6 and TNF-a, as well as inhibiting collagen synthesis [171]. As an alternative to tamoxifen chow, mouse studies have previously demonstrated that IP tamoxifen has little effect on weight [172]. Based on these observations, we revised our experimental design by including treatment with tamoxifen by IP injection. Tamoxifen IP injection demonstrated similar outcomes to tamoxifen chow, but without weight loss, allowing us to conclude that differences were due to tamoxifen.

While results between tamoxifen chow or daily tamoxifen IP injection are similar in females, there were several differences noted, mainly in effect size. These differences may be due to differences in bioavailability of tamoxifen for each dosing strategy, or by the differences in dosing between a controlled IP injection and an *ad libitum* diet of tamoxifen chow. In addition, there is the possibility that the weight loss seen in the tamoxifen chow group exhibited additional effects on top of the tamoxifen itself, potentiating some effects and antagonizing others.

It is relevant to note that, despite widespread clinical use, the mechanism of action of tamoxifen on biological systems is debated. While some studies have demonstrated direct effects through canonical estrogen receptor signaling pathways, separate studies have shown biological effects with no interaction through the canonical pathways [173-175]. It is likely that tamoxifen, as a steroid modulator, has multiple effects that can be enacted through a number of biological pathways within and outside of traditional canonical signaling. Additionally, tamoxifen has been shown to alter TGF-β signaling in some models, including differences in the TGF-β1 / TGF-β3 ratio. This is particularly relevant to tissue engineering, as fetal scarless healing is noted to have low TGF-β1 and high TGF-β3 [176]. Topical tamoxifen has seen some clinical success in reducing keloid scar formation, with a suggested mechanism of a reduction in TGF-β1 levels [177].

Despite tamoxifen's long-standing use in the laboratory as a Cre-Lox inducer and the prevailing thought that tamoxifen is essentially inert in the mouse model, multiple recent studies, including this one, have found confounding effects of tamoxifen on biological systems. In one study, tamoxifen IP injection in male mice attenuated CCL4-induced hepatotoxicity, downregulated CYP2E1 activity in the liver, and increased levels of antioxidants including catalase and superoxide dismutase. Tamoxifen also increased the presence of resident macrophages and recruitment of immune cells to necrotic areas of the liver [140]. IP tamoxifen increased browning of adipose tissue in female mice, but not male mice [172]. Careful consideration of these effects, and perhaps more that have not yet been elucidated, should be given when choosing to use tamoxifen in experimental models.

Overall, this study aims to demonstrate the complicated biological mechanisms at play in tissue engineering constructs. Even in syngeneic animals, the effects of sex cannot be ignored, and in fact can provide insight into important biological differences and potential avenues to improve tissue engineering outcomes. The use of any treatment on an animal or patient, in this case tamoxifen, can also have many unanticipated off-target effects on a tissue engineering system. The dosing route of the drug may also be an important factor in determining any confounding effects. Careful development of experimental design and thoughtful analysis of resulting outcomes will be crucial for the continued development of the field of tissue engineering, and determination of the biological mechanisms at play.

4. Methods

All surgeries, procedures, and experiments involving the use of animals in this study were done an accordance with relevant guidelines and regulations with approval from the Abigail Wexner Research Institute (AWRI) at Nationwide Children's Hospital Institutional Animal Care and Use Committee (IACUC) (Protocol AR12-00075). All animal experiments were performed in accordance with relevant guidelines and regulations and our animal study reporting adheres to the ARRIVE guidelines.

4.1 Scaffold Creation

Murine TEVGs were prepared as described previously[178]. Briefly, nonwoven polyglycolic acid (PGA) felt with a fiber diameter of 16μm was wound around a 19G needle to set the internal TEVG diameter, and inserted into a plastic mold to set the outer diameter. A 50:50 molar mixture of poly-L-lactide and poly-caprolactone (PCLA), 5% by mass/volume in dioxane was then used as a sealant for the TEVGs. Scaffolds were then frozen to -80C and lyophilized overnight to remove residual solvent.

4.2 Animal Treatments, TEVG Implantation, and Harvest

Male and female C57BL/6 mice aged 8-10 weeks were implanted with TEVGs as IVC interposition grafts using standard microsurgical techniques [95]. Briefly, after appropriate anesthesia with an intraperitoneal injection consisting of ketamine (100 mg/kg) and xylazine (10 mg/kg), a midline laparotomy incision was made, and a self-retaining retractor was inserted. The intestines were wrapped with gauze that was moistened in sterile saline. The aorta and IVC were separated, 2 microclamps were placed on the IVC, and the IVC was then transected between the microclamps. The graft was implanted as an IVC interposition graft with proximal and distal end-to-end anastomosis using a sterile 10-0 suture. Following skin closure, animals were moved to a recovery cage with a warming pad until they regained full mobility. Upon recovery, the mouse was returned to a new cage, and pain medication (ibuprofen) was provided in the drinking water for 48 h [179].

Tamoxifen was administered in chow (Envigo, Huntingdon, UK), beginning one week before implantation [135]. Mice were kept on the chow throughout the experimental study until endpoint. Mice were weighed on the day tamoxifen treatment began, the day of surgery, and the day of explant (POD 14).

To evaluate the administration route-specific effects of tamoxifen, an additional cohort of female mice was treated with 75 mg/kg body weight of tamoxifen dissolved in peanut oil by IP injection. Injections were done daily following the same timeline as the chow group in order to approximate the same dosing regimen.

A total of twenty mice were used per experiment group (male control, male tamoxifen chow, female control, female tamoxifen chow, female tamoxifen IP).

Two weeks after graft implantation (three weeks total after beginning tamoxifen treatment), mice were euthanized by deeply anesthetizing via intraperitoneal injection of an overdose of ketamine (200 mg/kg) and xylazine (20 mg/kg). Subsequently, the chest was cut open, and an incision was made on the right atrium; the mouse was systemically perfused from the left ventricle with 20 ml of 0.9% saline. Grafts were explanted surgically and divided in half, with one half being formalin fixed for histology, and the other half being snap-frozen in liquid nitrogen for RT-qPCR.

4.3 Histology

Explanted TEVG sections for histology were fixed overnight in formaldehyde at 4°C and transitioned to 70% ethanol. Sampled were then paraffin embedded and sectioned at 4μm. Samples were stained with H&E or Picro-Sirius Red, or left bare for immunohistochemistry. Immunohistochemistry sections were deparaffinized, rehydrated and blocked for endogenous peroxidase activity (3% H2O2 in H2O) and nonspecific background staining (3% normal goat serum in Background Sniper, BioCare Medical, CA, USA). Antigen retrieval was performed with citrate buffer (pH 6.0) or Tris-EDTA (pH 9.0) in a pressure cooker for 10 minutes and slides were incubated for 30 minutes at room temperature with primary antibodies. Primary antibodies included desmin (ab1520, abcam), CD31 (ab28364, abcam), CD68 (ab125212, abcam), Ki67 (ab15580, abcam), ER-α (ab271827, abcam), and ER-β (ab3576, abcam). Primary antibody binding was detected by subsequent incubation with species appropriate biotinylated IgG (Vector, CA, USA), followed by streptavidin-horse radish peroxidase (Vector) and chromogenic development with 3,3-diaminobenzidine (Vector). Tissue sections were counterstained with Gill's hematoxylin (Vector), and slides were dehydrated and cover slipped. Slides were imaged on a Zeiss Axio Observer Z1 inverted microscope (Zeiss, Germany) and quantified using ImageJ (NIH, USA). Images were de-identified and randomized prior to quantification to prevent bias. Collagen maturity was determined as percent of collagen fibers which demonstrated red/orange birefringence under polarized light.

4.4 Reverse Transcription Quantitative Real Time Polymerase Chain Reaction

Explanted TEVG sections were snap frozen and stored at -80C prior to transitioning to RNA*later*™-ICE (Invitrogen, AM7030) according to manufacture protocol. Samples were homogenized with a Qiagen Tissuelyser II and processed using an RNeasy Mini Kit (Qiagen, #74104). On column DNA digestion was performed with an RNase-Free DNase Set (Qiagen, #79254). Purified RNA was analyzed on a Nanodrop 2000c for concentration and 260/280 ratio greater than 1.8. Conversion of RNA to cDNA was performed with the High-Capacity RNA-to-cDNA kit (Applied Biosystems, #4388950). Custom-designed Taqman Array 96 well plates were used with the following hybridization (Taqman) probes: 18s rRNA (Hs99999901_s1), Actb (Mm02619580_g1), Hprt (Mm03024075_m1), B2m (Mm00437762_m1), Tgfb1 (Mm01178820_m1), Tgfb3 (Mm00436960_m1), NOS2 (Mm00440502_m1), Arg1 (Mm00475988_m1), Acta2 (Mm00725412_s1), S100a4 (Mm00803372_g1), Esr1 (Mm00433149_m1), Esr2 (Mm00599821_m1), Ccl2 (Mm00441242_m1), Mmp9 (Mm00442991_m1), F3 (Mm00438855_m1), and Igf1 (Mm00439560_m1). A gene maximation plate design was used loading equal amounts of cDNA for each sample with Taqman Fast Advanced Master Mix (Applied Biosystems, #4444556)[180]. Plates were run on an Applied Biosystems 7500 Real-Time PCR System. A total of 4 potential reference genes, 18srRNA, Actb, Hprt, and B2m, were run for every sample to determine the most stably expressed gene for the relative quantification. Resulting CT values for these 4 reference genes were analyzed utilizing the online tool

RefFinder, a combination of BestKeeper, NormFinder, Genorm, and the comparative Delta-Ct method [181]. B2m was determined to be the most stably expressed reference gene across all samples and was subsequently utilized for delta-delta CT relative quantification calculations.

4.5 Statistical Analysis

Data analysis was performed using GraphPad Prism 8.0 software (GraphPad, CA USA). Histology imaging for cellular markers was performed on 4 independent regions within each histological section, and averaged as technical replicates for comparison. RT-qPCR data was analyzed using delta-delta CT values, taken as the average of 2 technical replicates. Data was compared with t-tests between groups with experimental relevance (female control vs female tam chow, female control vs female tam IP, female control vs male control, male control vs male tam chow). Surgical survival and occlusion rate were compared using Fisher's exact test.

6. Figures

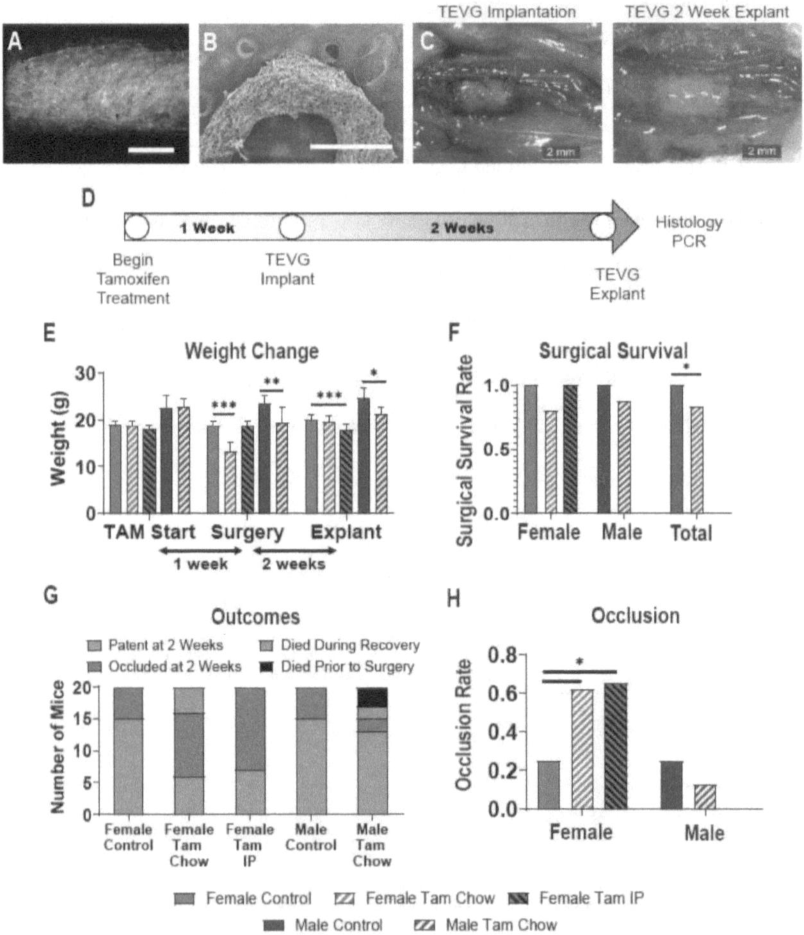

Figure 3-1 Experimental Overview and Outcomes

Transverse (A) and cross-sectional (B) view of the TEVG. C) TEVG at implantation (Left) and 2-week explantation (Right) as an IVC interposition graft. D) Timeline of tamoxifen treatment, implant, and explant. E) Survival and TEVG patency of all experimental animals. F) Surgical survival rate of mice on control diet, tamoxifen chow, and IP tamoxifen injection. G) Occlusion rate of TEVGs at 2-week explant. H) Weight of animals measured at tamoxifen start date, date of surgery, and explant at two weeks post-implantation. Scale bars = 500μm (A and B), 2mm (C). N = 15-20 for weight measurement and compared using t-tests. N = 15-20 for occlusion rate and compared using Fisher's exact test. *p<0.05, **p<0.01, ***p<0.001.

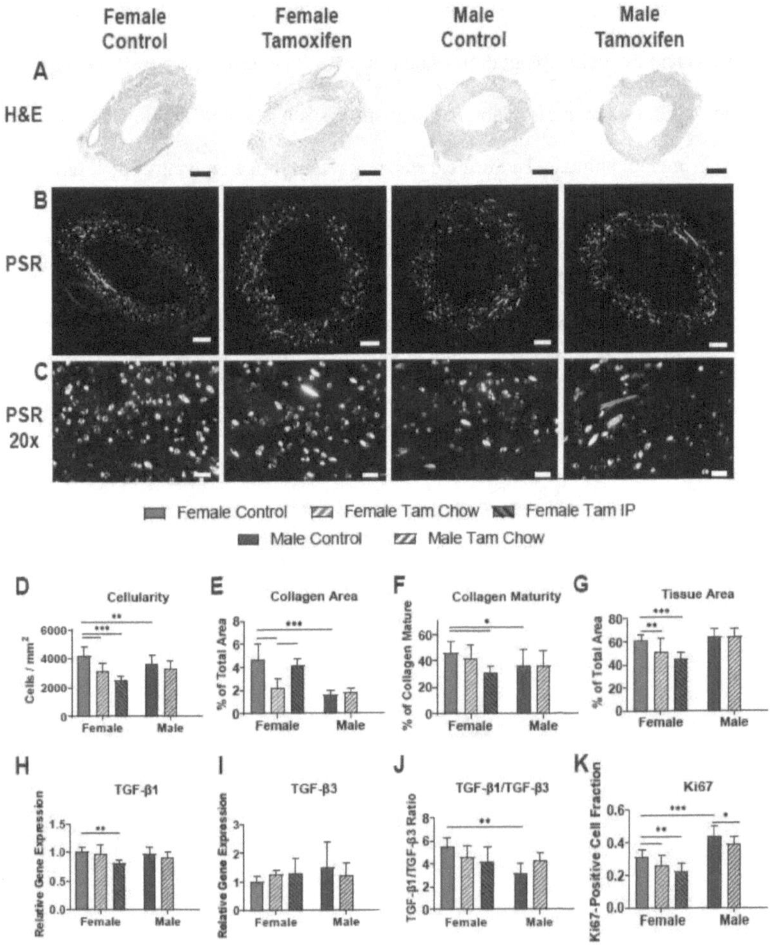

Figure 3-2 TEVG Neotissue Formation

A) H&E imaging of TEVGs at the 2-week time point. B) Picro-Sirius Red images under polarized light, with close-up of TEVG wall (C). White spots represent PGA fibers;

red/orange coloration represents mature thicker collagen fibers and yellow/green coloration represents thinner, immature collagen fibers, respectively. IHC quantifications of cellularity (D), tissue area (E), collagen area (F), collagen maturity (G), and Ki67 (H). RT-qPCR quantifications of TGF-β1 (I), TGF-β3 (J), and ratio of TGF-β1 to TGF-β3 (K). Scale bars = 0.5mm (A), 200μm (B) 20μm (C). N = 15-20 for histology measures (D-G), and N = 6 for RT-qPCR measures (H-K), all compared using t-tests. *p<0.05, **p<0.01, ***p<0.001.

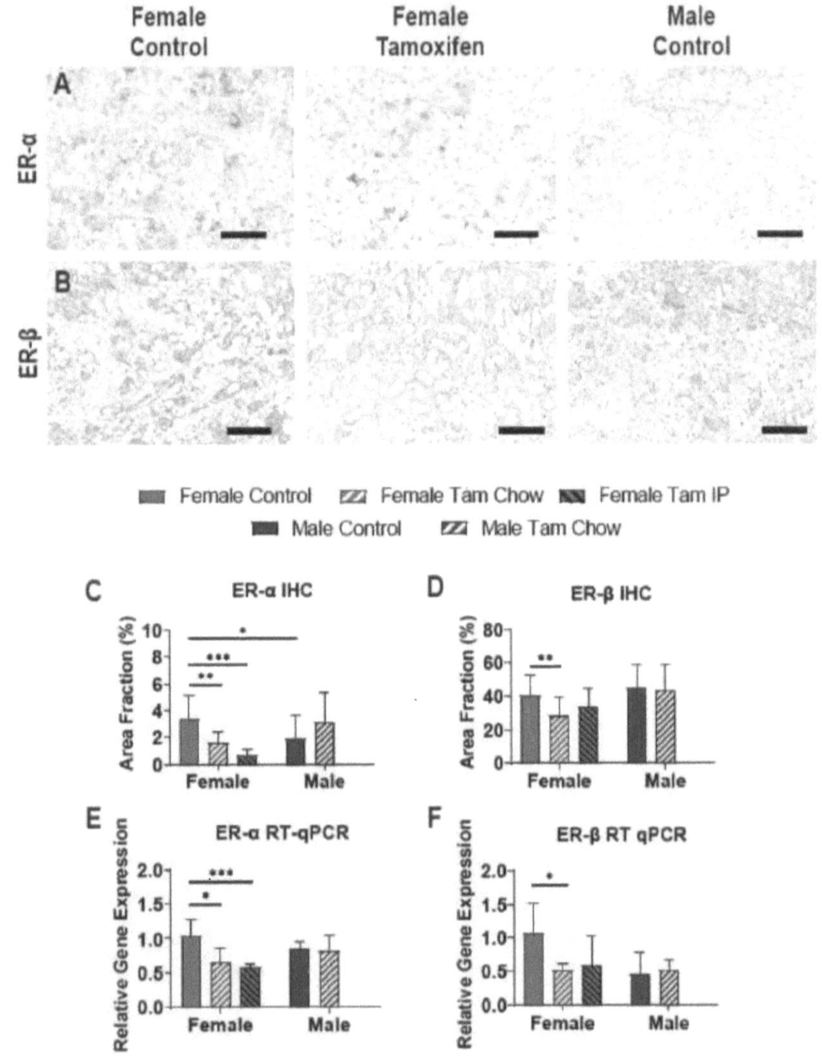

Figure 3-3 Estrogen Receptors Downregulated by Tamoxifen

Represenative IHC of ER-α (A) and ER-β (B). IHC quantifications of ER-α (C) and ER-β (D). RT-qPCR analysis of ER-α (E) and ER-β (F). N = 15-20 for histology measures (C, D), and N = 6 for RT-qPCR measures (E, F), all compared using t-tests. Scale bars = 200μm p<0.05, **p<0.01, ***p<0.001.

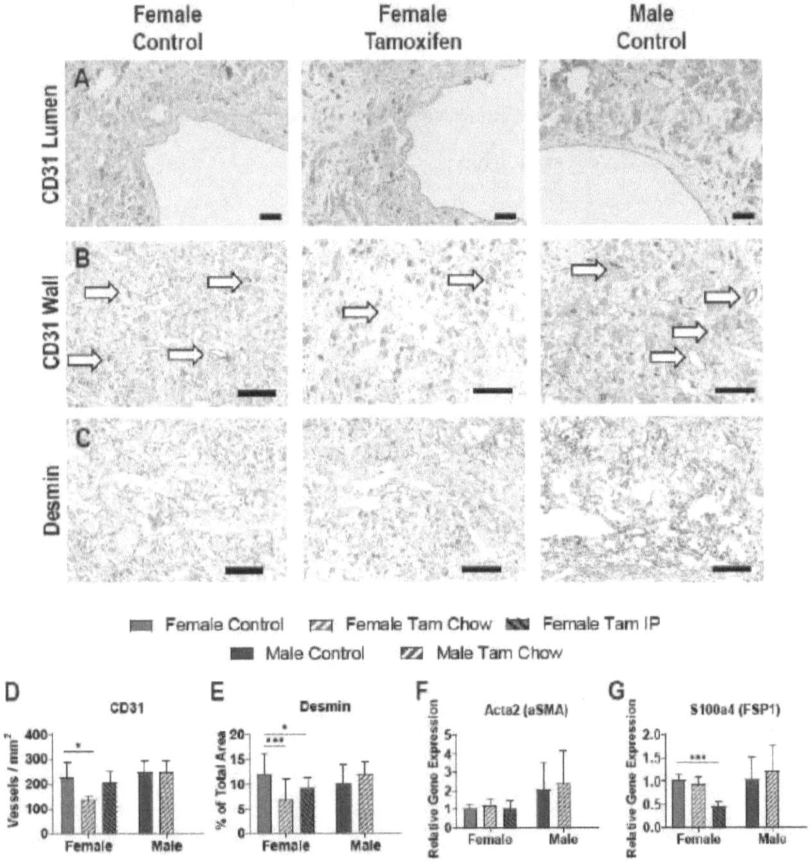

Figure 3-4 Tamoxifen Effects on Neotissue Cellular Make-Up

A) All TEVGs were endothelialized by 2 weeks as demonstrated by CD-31 staining. B) Walls of TEVGs contained vasa vasorum labeled with white arrows and quantified (D). C) Fibroblast and smooth muscle marker desmin staining shown within the TEVG wall and quantified (E). RT-qPCR quantification of acta2 (F) and S100a4 (G) Scale bars = 50μm

(A), 200μm (B and C). N = 15-20 for histology measures (D, E), and N = 6 for RT-qPCR measures (F, G), all compared using t-tests. *p<0.05, **p<0.01, ***p<0.001.

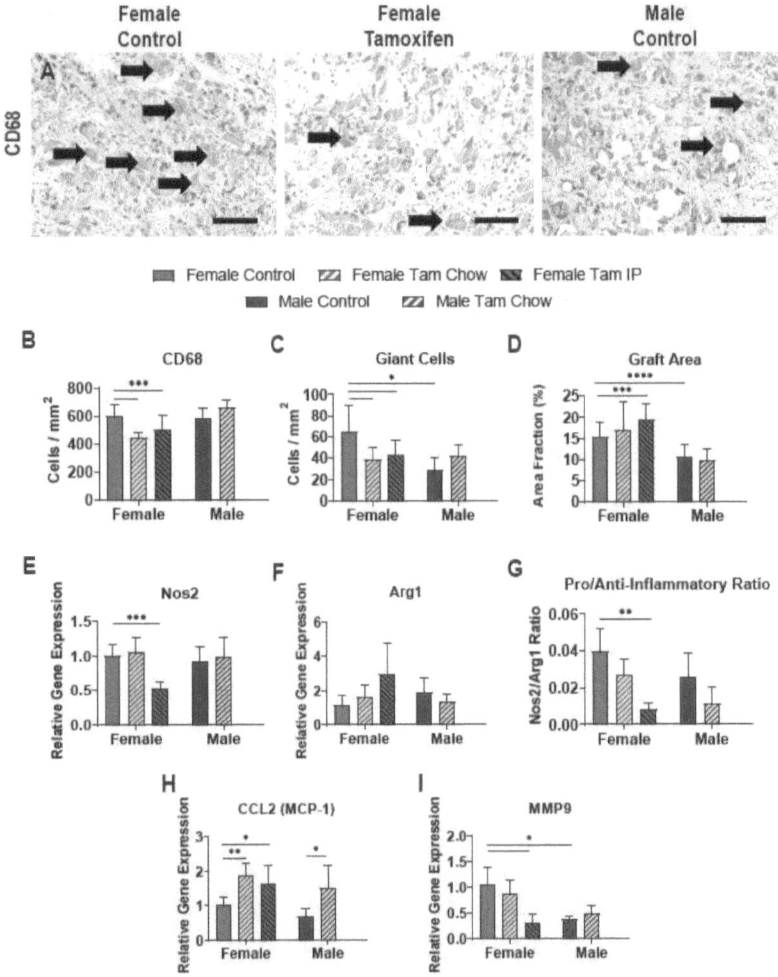

Figure 3-5 Tamoxifen Effects on Macrophage Response

A) Representative imaging of CD68 staining, with giant cells labeled with black arrows. Total CD68 positive cells quantified in (B) and giant cells quantified in (C). D) quantification of PGA polymer remaining in the wall of the TEVG 2 weeks after implantation. RT-qPCR quantification of pro-inflammatory NOS2 (E), anti-inflammatory Arg1 (F), and the ratio of the markers (G). RT-qPCR quantification of two markers of macrophage recruitment and function, CCL2 (H) and MMP9 (I). Scale bars = 200μm. N = 15-20 for histology measures (B-D), and N = 6 for RT-qPCR measures (E-I), all compared using t-tests. *$p<0.05$, **$p<0.01$, ***$p<0.001$

Chapter 4. An Analysis of the Natural History of Neovessel Formation in Tissue Engineered Vascular Grafts

1. Introduction

The development of a vascular conduit with growth potential holds great promise for advancing the field of congenital heart surgery where the risk of somatic overgrowth, the process of out-growing a synthetic graft and requiring additional surgery, is a significant concern [4, 182]. A promising solution to this problem is the use of tissue engineering methods to create a living vascular conduit that can grow with the patient, thus preventing somatic overgrowth [183]. Using tissue engineering methods, autologous vascular neotissue can either be generated *ex vivo* using a bioreactor-based approach and a patient's own cells or be created *in vivo* by implantation of a porous scaffold that allows for infiltration of host cells and removal of the scaffold [87]. Results of preclinical and clinical studies have confirmed the growth potential of TEVGs [65, 66]. Several different groups have developed tissue engineered vascular grafts (TEVG) specifically for this purpose [88, 184, 185]. The Xeltis Corporation has performed clinical trials using electrospun bioresorbable supramolecular polyester to create a vascular conduit for congenital heart surgery, with good results out to one year post-implantation [185]. The Tranquillo group has created vascular grafts using an *in vitro* approach to create decellularized tubes to implant as pulmonary arteries in sheep [186, 187]. The Niklason group utilized human vascular cells *in vitro* to create a tissue engineered vascular graft which was decellularized and implanted as hemodialysis access [188].

Despite significant advances in the development of this technology, there are currently no FDA-approved tissue engineered vascular grafts. We previously developed a TEVG designed specifically for use in children with congenital heart disease who require surgical implantation of a vascular conduit [64]. Our TEVG is made by seeding autologous bone marrow-derived cells onto a biodegradable tubular scaffold. Once seeded, the scaffold is implanted as a vascular conduit, where neotissue forms *in vivo* as the scaffold degrades. Interestingly, previous research has found that the seeded cells, rather than functioning as stem cells, serve a role in guiding neotissue formation through a paracrine mechanism [76]. The TEVG was utilized in a clinical trial for children with single ventricle disease as part of a modified Fontan operation, in which a vascular conduit is used to connect the inferior vena cava to the pulmonary artery [189]. Results of clinical trials evaluating this TEVG demonstrated an early period of dynamic remodeling ultimately resulting in the development of TEVG stenosis, which was successfully treated with angioplasty in patients who developed critical stenosis [65, 66, 190]. While all stenoses were ultimately treated successfully, its unexpected development has prevented FDA approval of the TEVG.

In order to improve our understanding of the processes underlying the formation of TEVG stenosis we developed a computational model of growth and remodeling which accurately predicted the formation of TEVG stenosis experienced in our clinical trial [66, 80]. The model is predicated on the mechano-biological behavior of native vessels, which respond to their hemodynamic environment in a predictable manner that can be modeled. Specifically, native vessels tend to exhibit a homeostatic set point, a predetermined amount of mechanical stress or strain that must be sensed by the cells in the vessel wall in order for the cells to be quiescent. In the short-term, vessels respond to deviations from the set point by vasoconstricting or vasodilating in order to alter hemodynamic forces to approach the set point. Chronic hemodynamic perturbation from the set point results in growth and remodeling of the vessel via inward or outward remodeling of the vessel lumen and thickening of the wall to alter wall circumferential stress and shear stress and attempt to restore mechanobiological homeostasis. Additionally, chronic hemodynamic perturbations from the set point can restore homeostasis by altering the thickness of the vessel wall to increase or decrease the amount of circumferential stress felt by cells within the vessel wall. The model suggested that TEVG stenosis is an inflammation-driven, mechano-mediated process and, unexpectedly, was likely to spontaneously reverse over time. We validated the model-generated hypothesis by testing this prediction using a large animal study that confirmed the reversible nature of TEVG stenosis [66].

Interestingly, the TEVG computational model is based on a model previously developed to describe and predict native vessel behavior, but modified to account for the biodegradable scaffold and its associated response [191]. Thus, the computational model suggests that once the scaffold is completely degraded the TEVG should transform into a neovessel that behaves like a native blood vessel. Herein, we confirm this model-generated hypothesis with an ovine inferior vena cava interposition model of the TEVG [192]. In this model, the TEVG is seeded with bone marrow-derived cells harvested on the day of surgery, and the TEVG is implanted as a thoracic IVC interposition graft. In previous studies, we demonstrated that the cells seeded onto scaffold do not directly contribute to and are not essential for neotissue formation, but do improve the performance of the TEVG by decreasing the incidence of TEVG stenosis [76].

We further investigate growth and remodeling of the TEVG using a hybrid computational-experimental approach to better understand the natural history of neovessel formation. Mathematical modeling of the TEVG was performed, and suggested the interconnected importance of mechanobiological and inflammatory cues in the development of TEVG neotissue. Juvenile lambs were implanted with TEVGs as thoracic IVC interposition grafts and followed for up to three years with serial angiography and intravascular ultrasound. Animals were sacrificed at predetermined timepoints for combinations of histology, mechanical testing, and vasoreactivity studies. Histological findings compared well with mathematical modeling predictions, and demonstrate that the TEVGs, after dynamic phases of neotissue formation and remodeling, develop into neovessels with native-like architecture and biological function, as well as native-like growth capacity.

2. Results

2.1 Natural history of neovessel formation

The scaffold is fabricated from polygylcolic acid (PGA) fibers that are knitted into a tube and coated with a 50:50 copolymer of polycaprolactone and polylactide (PCLA) which forms a porous sponge (**Figure 1A,B**). The scaffold is designed to degrade by hydrolysis over a period of 1 year. Initially upon implantation the scaffold functions as a synthetic vascular conduit. After implantation neotissue forms within and around the degrading scaffold. Neotissue formation in these TEVGs, as characterized by angiographic and histological measurements is consistently characterized by an early period of dynamic growth and remodeling over the first 6 months after implantation during which the TEVG undergoes dramatic morphometric changes resulting in graft narrowing during the first 6 weeks, followed by spontaneous dilation by 6 months. Beyond the initial 6-month period, changes in the morphometry of the TEVG are gradual, similar to native vessel growth and remodeling (**Figure 1C**). Once the scaffold is completely degraded the resulting structure, referred to as a neovessel, resembles a native blood vessel (**Figure 1D**).

2.2 Mechanisms underlying Growth and Remodeling

Intravascular ultrasound (IVUS) imaging over the 1 year time course demonstrates characteristic changes in the *in vivo* morphometry of the TEVG (**Figure 2A,B**), consistent with the angiographic measurements. Changes in size of the lumen of a conduit can arise from: (1) thickening or thinning of the wall of the graft, (2) inward or outward remodeling of the conduit lumen, or (3) combinations of both processes (**Figure 2C**). Serial IVUS data comparing wall thickness to luminal diameter demonstrated that between 1 and 6 weeks the lumen narrows primarily due to wall thickening through intramural growth. Imaging between 6 weeks and 6 months shows wall thinning in addition to inward remodeling, i.e. a decrease in outer diameter without a decrease in inner diameter. Between 6 months and 1 year the wall continues to thin, and the lumen expands (**Figure 2D,E**). Histological evaluation of the explanted grafts demonstrates that between 1 and 6 weeks after implantation, the luminal narrowing that causes TEVG stenosis is due primarily to scaffold wall thickening. The wall thickening arises from infiltration and proliferation of the scaffold-associated inflammatory cells, resulting in TEVG wall area at 6 weeks being 371±66% of the implanted scaffold wall area by IVUS. There is also evidence of appositional growth of vascular neotissue along the luminal surface of the scaffold, although it only accounts for 16±5% of total wall area at 6 weeks. Between 6 weeks and 6 months the TEVG stenosis spontaneously reverses as the wall thins. The thinning arises from degradation of the scaffold and loss of associated inflammatory neotissue, however the lumen is not completely restored to its preimplant area due to inward remodeling. Between 6 months and 1 year the wall thins further and expands the lumen as the scaffold and its associated inflammatory neotissue subside (**Figure 2D,E**).

2.3 Computational Model of Growth and Remodeling (G&R)

We previously developed and validated a computational model of growth and remodeling that accurately describes and predicts native vessel behavior (**Equation 1**) [66, 193]. Growth is defined as the change in mass of a tissue in response to a stimulus [194]. Remodeling is defined as the changes in microstructure, that result in changes to material behavior such as the anisotropy, stiffness and strength, e.g. matrix stiffening in fibrosis [195].

eq (1) Native tissue: $$\rho^{nat}(s) = \int_0^s m_h^{mech}\,(1 + \Upsilon^{mech}(\tau))q^{mech}(s,\tau)d\tau = \int_0^s M^{nat}(\tau)d\tau$$

eq (2) TEVG tissue: $$\rho^{neo}(s) = \rho^{infl}(s) + \rho^{mech}(s)$$

Mechano-mediated neotissue:

eq (3) $$\rho^{mech}(s) = \int_0^s M^{nat}(\tau)(1 - \exp(-\tau))\,d\tau$$

$$\rho^{mech}(s \to \infty) = \rho^{nat}(s)$$

Inflammation-mediated neotissue:

eq (4) $$\rho^{infl}(s) = \int_0^s m_h^{infl}\,(\Upsilon^{infl}(\tau))(1 - \exp(-\tau))q^{infl}(s,\tau)d\tau$$

$$\rho^{infl}(s \to \infty) = 0$$

$$\rho^{neo}(s \to \infty) = \rho^{mech}(s \to \infty) + \rho^{infl}\,(s \to \infty) = \rho^{nat}(s)$$

We subsequently modified and validated our computational model of growth and remodeling to describe and predict neotissue formation in TEVGs (**Equation 2**) [66]. The model was based on our original model describing native vessel growth and remodeling but with the addition of terms to describe and predict inflammation-mediated growth and remodeling induced by the TEVG scaffold, which we had previously demonstrated is critical to the process of neotissue formation. The computational model highlights the critical role the scaffold plays in determining TEVG behavior.

As the model has been shown to capture the physiologic TEVG neotissue formation data using a native vessel framework modified with inflammatory scaffold terms, we propose two important phenomenological predictions. The first prediction is that the scaffold should alter growth and remodeling via its stress shielding (**Equation 3**) and inflammation inducing characteristics (**Equation 4**). Of note, since the scaffold is biodegradable the scaffold properties and associated behavior, will change over time. Therefore, the behavior of the TEVG can be separated into two periods: the first period, hereafter referred to as the period of neotissue formation, during which the behavior is influenced by the presence of scaffold material and the second period, referred to as the period of neovessel remodeling, which occurs after scaffold degradation. The second model prediction is that after scaffold degradation, growth and remodeling of the neovessel should begin to mimic growth and remodeling in native vessels (**Equation 5**). This prediction is due to the mathematical framework of the TEVG growth and remodeling computational model, wherein after the scaffold has degraded, the equations will reduce to those used for modeling the native vasculature.

2.4 Role of the scaffold on growth and remodeling (*in vitro* degradation study)

Based on the computational model's prediction of the prominent role the scaffold plays on growth and remodeling in the TEVG, we characterized the properties of the scaffold that affect the inflammation-driven and mechano-mediated processes underlying neotissue formation. We characterized the mechanical properties of the scaffold including its compliance and burst pressure in order to determine the degree of stress shielding induced by the scaffold material. Since the scaffold is biodegradable, these characteristics of the scaffold change over time.

In order to determine how the inflammation-inducing and stress-shielding properties of the scaffold change over time, we performed an accelerated scaffold degradation study utilizing the temperature-dependent reaction kinetics of hydrolytic degradation of the polymers by bathing sections of the scaffold in PBS heated to 70°C *in vitro*. We analyzed specimens harvested over a time course (0, 1, 3, 5, 7, 9, and 14 days) (**Figure 3A-C**). Preliminary studies revealed that one day of accelerated degradation corresponded to 1 month of *in vivo* degradation (**Supplemental Figure**). Quantitative analysis of the accelerated scaffold degradation over time revealed complete degradation over 14 days but exhibited differential rates of polymer degradation with the PGA degrading by day 5 and the PCLA degrading by day 14 *in vitro* (**Figure 3D**). Morphometric characterization of the scaffold using SEM demonstrated that during degradation the pore size initially increased and then gradually decreased (**Figure 3E**) while the fiber diameter and alignment remained stable during the early period (0-5 days) but were dramatically altered as bulk erosion continued (7 days and beyond) (**Figure 3F**). After loss of mechanical integrity of the PCLA sponge, the scaffold material existed solely as floating pieces within the solution as it continued to degrade to the point of having no visible remaining pieces at 14 days.

Results of the degradation study demonstrate that the scaffold becomes progressively more compliant as it degrades (**Figure 3G**). There is a sudden increase of compliance (i.e. decrease in elastic modulus) at the 3-day time point corresponding with the loss of mechanical integrity of the PGA fibers (125±21 kPa day 0, 116±8 kPa day 1, 59±14 kPa day 3, day 1 vs day 3 t-test p value < 0.001) (**Figure 3H**). Similarly, the compliance increases to infinity (i.e. stiffness decreases to zero) as the PCLA sponge loses its mechanical integrity at 7 days *in vitro* (65±49 kPa day 5, 0±0 kPa day 7). Scaffold degradation demonstrates similar findings with respect to burst pressure, which drops precipitously at 3 days corresponding to loss of the PGA fiber integrity (>1000 kPa day 0 and day 1, 121±21 kPa day 3, 101±105 kPa day 5, 0±0 kPa day 7) and drops to a burst pressure of 0 mmHg at 7 days corresponding to loss of the PCLA sponge integrity (**Figure 3I**). Of note, from a physiologic perspective the scaffold remains relatively stiff compared to the native IVC over the physiologically relevant pressure range (1-20 mm Hg) until after

5 days of accelerated degradation. Finally, results of the *in vitro* degradation study demonstrate an uncoupling of the change in the inflammation inducing properties of the scaffold and the stress shielding properties of the scaffold since the loss of stress shielding occurs long before the full mass of the scaffold has degraded.

2.5 Role of the scaffold on growth and remodeling (in vivo time course study)

Next we evaluated scaffold induced inflammation *in vivo*. We performed a time course experiment, evaluating the performance of the TEVG in an ovine IVC vascular interposition graft model. We harvested the grafts at 1, 6, 26, and 52 weeks after implantation and characterized the grafts using immunohistochemical (IHC) stains (**Figure 4A**). Markers of the inflammatory response, including CD45 for non-specific leukocytes and CD68 for monocytes and macrophages were present within the neotissue formed within the scaffold. Histological evaluation of the explanted grafts demonstrated that the degradation of the scaffold *in vivo* mirrored its degradation *in vitro*, including differential rates of polymer degradation with the PGA fibers (solid black) degrading prior to the PCLA (black outline) between the 6-week and 6-month time point (**Figure 4B**). However, histological analysis of the scaffold degradation also demonstrated some scattered residual scaffold material and areas of inflammatory cells still present at the 52 week time point revealing that some differences do exist between polymer degradation *in vivo* and *in vitro*. Another important finding was that the thickness of the scaffold material increased from the manufactured thickness of 0.70 mm at implant to 1.32±0.25 mm at 1-week and 2.97±0.64 mm at the 6-week time point (1 week vs 6 week t-test p value < 0.001) then narrowed to 1.86±0.39 mm by the 6-month time point (6 week vs 6 month t-test p value <

0.001). As this thickening did not occur with scaffold immersion in fluid *in vitro*, it is likely related to the infiltration and extracellular matrix deposition of inflammatory cells following scaffold implantation.

The IHC staining revealed populations of inflammatory cells within the wall of the scaffold throughout the remodeling time course. CD45-positive leukocyte cell populations, including CD68-positive monocytes and macrophages, are rapidly drawn into the scaffold, populating the porous structure. The inflammatory stimulus, measured by CD45+ cells, continued to mount a response to a peak around 6 weeks (437±91 cells/mm), after which the inflammatory cell populations decreased over time (257±110 cells/mm^2 at 26 weeks, t-test vs 6 weeks $p < 0.001$), becoming closer to, but still higher than, the native background inflammatory cell population by 1 year (148±63 cells/mm^2 TEVG vs 34±28 cells/mm^2 IVC; 26 week TEVG vs 1 year TEVG t-test p value 0.011; 1 year TEVG vs IVC t-test p value <0.001). Pro-inflammatory (iNOS positive) and anti-inflammatory (CD163 positive) macrophages and monocytes appear to rise and fall in tandem over the course of the TEVG neotissue evolution. At one year, there were slightly higher levels of lingering anti-inflammatory macrophages compared to pro-inflammatory macrophages (31±21 iNOS+ cells/mm^2 vs 65±34 CD163+ cells/mm^2, t-test p value = 0.008), likely related to long-term retention of low levels of foreign body giant cells within the neotissue.

We also evaluated the effect of the *in vivo* stress shielding properties of the scaffold. *Ex vivo* biaxial mechanical testing of neovessels (**Figure 5A**) demonstrated that at the early 6-week time point, when inflammation and wall thickness are high and a large amount of the scaffold remains, the TEVG is much stiffer than the native IVC, demonstrating lower axial stress (1.54±0.58 kPa 6 week vs 11.72±0.56 kPa 18 month vs 16.80 kPa IVC) (**Figure 5B**), circumferential stress (8.50±3.00 kPa 6 week vs 58.99±2.20 kPa 18 month vs 71.56 kPa IVC) and distensibility (0.0018±0.0008 mm/mmHg 6 week vs 0.0068±0.0021 mm/mmHg 18 month vs 0.0128 mm/mmHg IVC) than the native IVC at *in vivo* stretch and representative pressures. At 18 months post implantation, distensibility, axial and circumferential stress approach native IVC values. The *in vivo* stretch and circumferential stretch are however lower than the native IVC, suggestive of an altered matrix composition. The biomechanical properties of the TEVG arise from the combination of the mechanical properties of the scaffold and the biomechanical properties of the neotissue, which are derived primarily from the deposited extracellular matrix (ECM). Immediately after implantation, biomechanical properties of the TEVG are derived exclusively from the mechanical properties of the scaffold, but over time they transition to the properties of the deposited extracellular matrix. At long time points when the scaffold is absent and neovessel formation is complete, mechanical behavior for the graft is exclusively derived from the ECM. Evaluation of the stress shielding properties of the scaffold *in vivo* are consistent with the *in vitro* characterization and demonstrate that up to the 6-week time point the TEVG is stiff relative to the native IVC but over the course of a year, as the scaffold degrades the TEVG becomes more compliant approaching the compliance of the native IVC.

Evaluation of the ECM demonstrates significant remodeling and maturation over time from a disordered structure to a highly ordered structure, which proceeds with the loss of stress shielding and the initiation of mechano-mediated growth and remodeling. Histological analysis of the structurally significant constituents in the neotissue revealed similar findings (**Figure 5C,D**). The total area of neotissue increased up to 6 weeks (12.7 mm^2 1 week vs 138.0±37.7 mm^2 6 week), when the inflammatory status peaked, and then decreased as the inflammation subsided and the stenosis self-resolved (65.4±31.9 mm^2 26 week vs 30.3±11.2 mm^2 52 week, t-test p value = 0.003). After implantation, the cellular content of the TEVG was high (81%) and the collagen content was low (19%) as measured by trichrome staining. This ratio reverses over time, at one year approaching the low cellularity, high collagen content of the native IVC (78.8±6.6% TEVG vs 91.3±4.8% IVC trichrome collagen area, t-test p value < 0.001). Notably, by picrosirius red staining, the collagen content at 1 year in the TEVG was not different from that of the native IVC (85.0±10.6% 1 year TEVG vs 86.5±8.0% IVC PSR collagen area, t-test p value = 0.649) The ratio of thick collagen I fibers to thinner collagen III fibers changes as the TEVG neotissue evolves, with type I collagen becoming a significantly larger proportion of the total collagen at later time points. However, the ratio remains lower than that seen in the native IVC at one year (23.5±8.5 TEVG vs 43.3±52.2 IVC, thick vs thin collagen ratio, t-test p value = 0.224), although there was much variation in the ratios of native IVC samples.

2.6 Fluid Dynamic Changes

eNOS staining for endothelial cells demonstrated little to no staining at 1 week, disconnected staining along the lumens of the TEVGs at 6 weeks, and complete luminal staining at 26 weeks and beyond, appearing similar to the endothelial staining along the lumen of the native IVC (**Figure 6A**). Reconstructions of MRI evaluations of TEVGS at 1 week, 6 weeks, and 1 year post-implantation (**Figure 6B**) coupled with computational fluid dynamics modeling demonstrated the characteristic changes seen in the natural history of TEVG neotissue formation and development, including the development of focal stenosis and subsequent fluid jet at 6 weeks, with resolution by one year. Quantifications of area and wall thickness demonstrate similar findings along the length of the TEVG (**Figure 6C,D**). Shear stress (**Figure 6E**) was seen to increase from 1 to 6 weeks, particularly in the area of stenosis, with less variation in shear stress seen along the TEVG at one year, which showed steady shear stress along the length at a notably higher level than the 1 week TEVG. Cauchy stress (**Figure 6F**) showed large increases from 1 to 6 weeks, with decreases back to one week levels by one year post-implantation.

2.7 Computational Analysis of Inflammation driven, mechano-mediated neotissue formation

Previous clinical studies and computational simulations demonstrated that the TEVGs were prone to early stenosis, which would spontaneously resolve over time as the balance of immunological and mechanobiological stimuli shifted, while the scaffold degrades and neotissue forms (**Figure 7A**). With this framework, we probed the importance of these mechanisms by demonstrating *in silico* the effects of eliminating each stimulus. When the immune response to the scaffold was muted, the TEVG demonstrated early rapid dilation due to a lack of early neotissue formation as the scaffold degraded. Over time, the development of mechano-mediated neotissue led to progressive narrowing of the TEVG towards the original diameter. On the other hand, by including only immuno-mediated matrix production early events of TEVG growth and remodeling were still observed, namely the early stenosis followed by resolution, but the lack of mechano-mediated matrix production led to substantial dilatation of the graft at late time points as the immuno-mediated matrix degraded without new native matrix production to replace it. These simulations highlight the importance of both inflammation- and mechano-mediated neotissue formation on TEVG behavior.

We extracted the relative contribution of the inflammation-driven and mechano-mediated constituents on neotissue growth and remodeling over the simulated 1 year time course, which demonstrated that neotissue formation is primarily inflammation driven during the first 6 months after implantation and then rapidly transitions to mechano-mediated after 6 months (**Figure 7B**). These findings compare well with trends seen in our experimental degradation and histological data (**Figure 7C,D**) that suggest that during the first 6 weeks neotissue formation is exclusively driven by inflammation. This results in luminal narrowing due to wall thickening composed primarily of inflammatory tissue within the wall of the scaffold. Between 6 weeks and 6 months the degree of inflammation-driven neotissue formation decreases as the scaffold degrades, resulting in wall thinning and causing an increase in luminal size. However, this is partially offset by the initiation of mechano-mediated remodeling as the scaffold becomes more compliant and loses its stress shielding capacity, resulting in inward remodeling. Between 6 months and 1 year, as the scaffold finishes degrading, inflammation-driven neotissue formation continues to diminish resulting in further wall thinning which is augmented by the mechano-mediated growth and remodeling as the ECM matures and the neovessel wall becomes more compliant and the lumen expands while the wall thins.

In comparing our computational modeling predictions of inflammatory neotissue and mechanical neotissue to our explanted histology, we find strong agreement. There were slight differences seen, notable in the histological mixture of mechanical and inflammatory neotissues being similar at 26 weeks, while the modeled crossing was seen at approximately 36 weeks after implantation. *In vivo* measurements also demonstrated a longer-lasting inflammatory response than that seen in the modeling predictions (**Figure D**).

The relative contributions and relationship between inflammation-driven and mechano-mediated growth and remodeling were further demonstrated by correlating our morphometric and IHC data over time which reveal a significant positive correlation between iNOS and intramural growth (linear regression $p < 0.0001$, $R^2=0.628$) which supports the model-based prediction of inflammation-mediated luminal narrowing and our experimental data demonstrating that this is due to inflammation-driven wall thickening. In addition, there was also a significant correlation between calponin and inward remodeling (linear regression $p = 0.0023$, $R^2=0.278$) supporting the model prediction of mediation of geometric changes by mechano-sensitive smooth muscle cells and our experimental data demonstrating the role of inward remodeling on the remodeling of stenosis between 6 weeks and 6 months after implantation.

2.8 Neovessels resemble native vessels in structure and function

Our computational model formulation suggests that after scaffold degradation, growth and remodeling of the TEVG neovessel should be similar to growth and remodeling in native vessels. At one year post implantation, surface SEM demonstrated a contiguous surface covering of endothelial cells, and *en face* staining of the luminal surface with CD31 and eNOS suggested the presence of a competent endothelium (**Figure 8A**). IHC analysis of the neovessel compared to the native vessel demonstrated that the neovessel has a thin laminated wall composed of an intima, media and adventitia similar to the native IVC (**Figure 8B**). The intima is composed of a monolayer of CD31+ endothelial cells surrounded by concentric layers of calponin+ smooth muscle cells. Time course immunohistochemical studies reveal that calponin+ smooth muscle cells increased rapidly from 6 to 26 weeks (0.021±0.014 6-week vs 0.060±0.015 26-week Calponin+ area fraction, t-test p value < 0.001), after which the levels remained similar to that seen in the native IVC (**Figure 8C**) (0.055±0.020 52-week TEVG vs 0.050±0.019 IVC, Calponin+ area fraction, t-test p value $= 0.485$). When examining the total amount of Calponin+ area, the amount increased from 1 to 6 weeks, stayed steady to 26 weeks before reducing to a lower area at 52 weeks as the neovessel matured.

To further characterize neovessel functionality, we subjected several long-term implants (>1.5 years) to vasoreactivity testing (**Figure 8D-G**). Results demonstrated that the TEVG neovessel has similar contractile responses to that of the native IVC for both KCL and endothelin-1 (**Figure 8D,E**). Although not statistically different from the native IVC, the TEVG did not experience as much relaxation to acetylcholine (**Figure 8F**). The relaxation response to SNP was also similar to that of the native IVC (**Figure 8G**). Together, these results suggest the development of native-like structure and function.

2.9 Neovessels exhibit biological growth

In addition to investigating neotissue deposition and remodeling into functional neovessels, we sought to evaluate the biological growth potential of the TEVG. Biological growth refers to the progressive change in size, shape, and function that occurs as a result of the development and maturation of an organism. We implanted the TEVG in juvenile lambs in order to evaluate their biological growth potential as they matured to adult sheep (**Figure 9A**). The lambs more than doubled in weight during the first year following implantation (26.8±3.8 Kg 1-week, 64.2±5.5 Kg 1 year, t-test p value < 0.001) and continued to grow steadily out to two years before leveling off in weight (79.6±9.2Kg 2-year, 76.8±11.2Kg 3-year, t-test p value = 0.446) (**Figure 9B**). In comparing our implanted animals to age matched non-implanted controls, we found that our implanted animals had similar growth, suggesting that the TEVG implant in the IVC did not cause any growth restriction of the animal.

Volumetric reconstructions based on serial 3D angiography of the TEVG demonstrated that the TEVG lumen underwent an initial decrease in volume reaching its nadir at 6 weeks after implantation (3.6±0.9 mL 1 week vs 1.8±0.9 mL 6 week, t-test p value < 0.001) then increasing in volume over the ensuing 150-week period (3.5±1.3 mL 26 week vs 5.0±2.5 mL 156 week, t-test p value = 0.018) (**Figure 9C,D**). The caudal IVC next to the TEVG, measured from the suture line of the TEVG to the site of the surgical cannulation clip, was utilized as an internal control. This region was shown to grow rapidly over the first 6 months (1.22±0.65 mL 1 week vs 2.83±0.63 mL 6 weeks, 3.63±0.45 mL 6 months), before decreasing to 1 year and then continuing to grow after this point (2.33±0.76 mL 1 year,

3.22±0.79 mL 2 years, 3.42±1.56 mL 3 years). This counter-intuitive trend can be explained by considering the pressure build up due to the TEVG stenosis, which expanded the native IVC until the stenosis resolved. Notably, from 1 to 3 years the rates of growth of the TEVG and the caudal IVC were similar. During the same period of time TEVG became progressively more compliant. Comparison of the area deformation of the TEVG and IVC over the cardiac cycle by MRI revealed that upon implantation the TEVG was relatively stiff compared to the IVC at one week (0.24±0.08 IVC vs 0.10±0.02 TEVG, fractional area deformation, Mann-Whitney test p value < 0.0001), but by one-year post-implantation the neovessel appeared to pulse similarly to the surrounding native IVC (0.23±0.12 IVC vs 0.26±0.06 TEVG, fractional area deformation, Mann-Whitney test p value = 0.400) (**Figure 9E,F**). This increase in compliance is important to consider, because the IVC is a highly compliant vessel that changes its volume dramatically based on the hemodynamic forces, which allows it to serve its function as a capacitance vessel. Thus, assessing growth based on volume or diameter alone could be confounded by differences in the hemodynamic states of an animal at different time points. In contrast, the length of a vessel is not effected by the hemodynamic state and therefore represents a better measure of biological growth capacity. Thus, we measured the change in TEVG length over time and compared it to the change in vertebral body height measured on the same angiogram. Serial measurements revealed that the TEVG initially decreased in length during the first 6 weeks (21.4±2.2 mm 1 week 18.1±3.1 mm 6 week, t-test p value = 0.001) then subsequently increased in length (21.0±4.1 mm 26 week vs 28.3±2.3 mm 156 week, t-test p value < 0.001) at a rate similar to the rate of change in height to the vertebral body

(21.7±1.6 mm 26 week vs 27.12±2.4 mm 156 week) over the ensuing time course (**Figure 9G**).

3. Discussion

In this study, we used an integrative computational-experimental approach to investigate the natural history of growth and remodeling in TEVG. Growth and remodeling were simulated using a constrained mixture model which was based on a previously validated computational model developed for describing and predicting growth and remodeling in native vessels [66, 80]. The model highlighted the critical role the scaffold plays in inducing inflammation-driven neotissue formation and mechano-mediated remodeling (**Figure 7A,D**). The model-based predictions suggested we focus our study on evaluating how the inflammation-inducing and stress-shielding properties of the biodegradable scaffold change over time and induce and modulate neotissue formation *in vivo*. Results of our computational-experimental studies provide valuable insights into dynamic changes that occur during the first 6 months after TEVG implantation during which the scaffold degrades. Furthermore, our model suggested that after scaffold degradation the resulting neovessel should exhibit growth and remodeling which mimics the behavior of native vessels. Together these findings provide insights into development and translation, and have important implications for the use of the TEVG to the clinic.

Previous studies by our group have demonstrated that cell seeding is not essential for neovessel formation but does modulate outcomes [196-198]. We have shown that the cells seeded onto the TEVG scaffold disappear shortly after implantation and do not directly give rise to the vascular neotissue, as has been noted for many stem cell-related therapies in recent years [199-202]. Instead we have discovered that inflammation, which is induced by implantation of the scaffold, is essential for neotissue formation [75, 203, 204]. Depletion of the monocytes and macrophages using either clodronate liposomes or diphtheria toxin (using a transgenic DT CD11b mouse model) block vascular neotissue formation [75]. Results of cell tracking and cell lineage tracing experiments demonstrate that the endothelial cells and smooth muscle cells that give rise to the intimal and medial layers of the neovessel arise from the neighboring vessel wall [77]. Thus, the monocytes and macrophages that infiltrate the scaffold induce the ingrowth of endothelial cells and smooth muscle cells along the surface of the scaffold via IL-10 and MCP-1 dependent paracrine signaling mechanisms [205]. We have previously shown that the phenotype of the infiltrating macrophages plays a critical role in neotissue formation [134, 157, 203]. Interestingly the macrophage that infiltrate the scaffold exhibit both pro-inflammatory and anti-inflammatory markers and the relative percentage of these cells remains constant throughout the process of neovessel formation (**Figure 4B**). This inflammatory-driven process is reminiscent of what occurs in lower order species which possess the ability to regenerate in that the regenerative process can be blocked by clondronate liposomes and that the inflammatory cells simultaneously exhibit a mixed phenotype which drives the regenerative process [206-208].

While inflammation is essential for neovessel formation, excessive inflammation leads to the formation of TEVG stenosis. Previous studies demonstrate that cell seeding reduces the incidence of the formation of TEVG stenosis by altering the foreign body reaction to the scaffold via a TGF-β paracrine mechanism [123, 157]. Similarly, we have demonstrated that the monocytes that infiltrate the scaffold arise from the splenic reservoir and their release into the circulation is controlled by angiotensin I receptor [75, 209]. Results of this current study demonstrate that in the ovine IVC vascular interposition graft model inflammation peaks at around 6 weeks and decreases thereafter as the scaffold degrades. The bulk of the wall thickening that leads to the early TEVG stenosis arises from accumulation of inflammatory cells as the scaffold thickens during the degradation process. The subsequent wall thinning that occurs between 6 weeks and 6 months after implantation is due to the resolution of the foreign body reaction as the scaffold material is resorbed and degraded.

Previously we had postulated that growth and remodeling experienced in our clinical studies were flow-dependent phenomena. The computational model lends further credence to this hypothesis. The inclusion of terms describing mechano-mediated growth and remodeling are essential for accurately describing and predicting the growth and remodeling experienced in our experimental studies. During the first 6 months after implantation, the scaffold provides a significant stress shielding effect to the neotissue since the scaffold remains noncompliant at the level of the hemodynamic forces exerted by the flow of blood through the IVC conduit. By 6 months after implantation, the stress shielding effect of the scaffold has dissipated due to scaffold degradation with the exception of a few scattered fragments, which are no longer connected enough to carry the physiologic stresses within the neovessel wall. Scaffold mechanics have been previously shown to have large effects on neotissue formation *in vivo* [98, 210, 211]. However, as the scaffold degrades and the stress-shielding properties of the scaffold diminish, the role of mechano-mediated remodeling becomes more prominent. Beyond the 6-month period after implantation when the scaffold is degraded, growth and remodeling become mechano-driven and can be well described through maintenance of mechanical homeostasis. During this period not only does the extracellular matrix remodel to better resemble the compliance and stress state of the native IVC (**Figure 2**) but the neovessel also becomes vasoreactive (**Figure 8D-F**), enabling it to respond to alterations in the hemodynamic environment. Endothelialization of the TEVG was found to occur by the 6 month implant time point, with sparse endothelial cells seen at 6 weeks (**Figure 6**). This finding further supports the computational modeling prediction that flow-mediated and mechanical signals are dominated by the inflammatory signals at early time points, as the neotissue lacks a functional endothelium to sense and respond to the flow. Previous research has shown a severe limitation of endothelialization distance along vascular grafts, however the unique environment of each individual graft, in particular the effects of degradable scaffolds, is important to consider for endothelialization as well as other phenomena of remodeling [212, 213].

The computational model describes the complex interplay between inflammation and mechano-mediated neotissue formation which can be difficult to predict intuitively. For example, during the first 6 weeks after implantation, growth and remodeling are essentially exclusively inflammation-mediated due the extreme degree of stress shielding. Growth and remodeling are determined by wall thickening due to the natural progression of the foreign body reaction which occurs in a reproducible and predictable manner. Similarly, beyond the 6-month period after scaffold degradation, when neovessel behavior is determined by mechano-mediated processes, change occurs more gradually and in a more native vessel-like manner. During the time period between 6 weeks and 6 months, the interplay between these mechanisms is dynamic and complex since the inflammation-mediated effects change as the scaffold degrades and directly impact the mechano-mediated remodeling by altering the biomechanical characteristics of the wall of the vessel and the hemodynamic forces exerted on the vessel. The interaction between these mechanisms results in wall thinning that is partly counteracted by inward remodeling. The net result is the reversal of the inflammation-mediated TEVG stenosis but not to the luminal size of the original TEVG implant.

The computational model sheds additional light on biological growth potential of the TEVG since native mechano-mediated processes are inhibited by the early immune response. Thus, the growth capacity of the TEVG should be evaluated in this study starting after the loss of stress shielding, which in this study was at the 6 month post implantation period. The model also suggests that there are at least two phases to consider based on the presence or absence of the scaffold. During the first phase, the period of neotissue formation, the scaffold lacks normal biological growth potential. This is particularly noticeable during the first 6 weeks after implantation when neotissue formation is primarily inflammation-driven due to the presence of the scaffold which restricts growth (**Figure 2, Figure 9**). After the 6-week time point when the scaffold loses its biomechanical integrity due to polymer degradation, growth is no longer restricted. However, the presence of the inflammatory residual scaffold material continues to affect growth and remodeling until it is more fully degraded by the 6 month period and beyond.

An important benefit to our computational-experimental approach used here is the ability for computational studies to guide relevant experimentation, and the ability of experimental results to update and refine the computational model. As the material and mechanical properties of the scaffold are the guiding forces of inflammation and neotissue formation in the early time points, computational modeling can be beneficial in navigating the potential scaffold parameter space *in silico* [96]. Coupled with guided *in vivo* experimentation around the edges of this parameter space, this computational-experimental approach can suggest key time points and scaffolding parameters for evaluation, and experimental results can be compared and contrasted with modeling outcomes to determine new effects and interactions to create a more accurate model [95, 102, 210]. This method has the benefit of decreasing the needed number of animals for experimentation, and may accelerate new design development through the suggestion of optimized scaffold parameters.

One of the limitations of our computational model in its current form is that it is not designed to describe or predict individual graft performance but instead describe the mean behavior of the group. Thus, growth and remodeling for any individual TEVG may deviate significantly from the model based predictions. As we move forward and continue to develop the model, our predictive capabilities would be benefitted by creating a fluid-solid growth model that will meld our fluid and solid models. This fluid-solid-growth model may be informed with patient specific hemodynamics, thereby improving its ability to predict growth and modeling behavior relative to the individual. Similarly, recent work using targeted molecular imaging to quantify an individual's foreign body reaction to the

TEVG scaffold can be used to inform the computational model thereby improving its ability to describe and predict the *in vivo* behavior of an individual's TEVG [79]. This approach could open the door to adopting personalized medicine approach for managing patients after implantation of the TEVG.

Results of our study utilizing a computational-experimental approach to investigate the natural history of neovessel formation highlighted the critical role of the scaffold on determining growth and remodeling, and therefore *in vivo* performance, of the TEVG. Ultimately the computational model can be used to perform optimization studies designed to refine the design and improve the performance of the TEVG. Based on the results of this study several characteristics of the scaffold were identified which could potentially be modified to improve the performance of the TEVG. The first is the uncoupling of the inflammation and mechano-mediating properties of the scaffold. This results in formation of early TEVG narrowing as inflammation drives the formation of neotissue within the wall of the thick, stiff scaffold. The second scaffold characteristic identified is the sudden loss of stress shielding which occurs as the scaffold transforms from being relatively stiff to highly compliant. This sudden change in the mechanical properties of the scaffold arises from the breaking of degrading polymer fibers resulting in loss of the integrity of the scaffold. A more gradual transition could minimize the dynamic changes in growth and remodeling exhibited during the first 6 months after implantation. The third scaffold property to be optimized is the degradation process. The scaffold is designed to degrade by hydrolysis, which allows for analysis of degradation *in vitro*. Results of this study confirm differences in the rate of degradation *in vivo* that manifest themselves by heterogeneous distribution of small amounts of residual polymer in specimens implanted beyond the 6-month time period. Though limited in amount, these materials serve as a persistent source of inflammation and mechanical-shielding which can impact growth and remodeling. More homogenous and complete degradation *in vivo* would be optimal.

Autologous biological vascular conduits significantly outperform other synthetic or biological grafts [87]. Unfortunately, the amount of autologous vascular tissue available for performing major cardiovascular reconstructive procedures is quite limited, necessitating the use of synthetic or non-autologous biomaterials for most major congenital heart operations. Use of these biomaterials results in significant morbidity and mortality. The fundamental premise underlying the development of a TEVG is that it would provide a method for creating an increased supply of autologous vascular tissue for surgical reconstruction. Herein we have demonstrated that the TEVG transforms into a neovessel that behaves like a native vessel, however; with some caveats due to performance issues related to growth and remodeling which occurs during the first 6 months after implantation. Herein we demonstrate that the neovessel possesses biological growth potential, however the biologic growth potential of the TEVG is only realized after the scaffold has degraded and the neovessel has formed. Prior to neovessel formation the neotissue undergoes dynamic remodeling resulting in an initial net loss in lumen size compared the size of the scaffold upon implantation. Similarly, the neovessel develops the attributes of a native vessel including the formation of a functional endothelial layer and the formation of a highly compliant and vasoreactive wall which matches the compliance and vasoreactivity of the vessel into which it is implanted. The development of these biomimetic properties have important implications for optimizing the long-term performance of these grafts, especially when used in the pediatric population. Moving forward, continued utilization of a computational-experimental approach holds great promise for improving our understanding of the mechanisms underlying neovessel formation which in turn can be used to direct their use, optimize their design and improve their performance in a time and cost-efficient manner.

4. Methods

4.1 Mathematical Modeling

Growth and remodeling of TEVGs was simulated using a constrained mixture theory growth and remodeling framework outlined in detail previously [66]. Briefly, the mass density of each structurally significant wall constituent, including smooth muscle cells and collagen fibers, were tracked through the remodeling course via a series of quasi-equilibrated time steps. The mass densities of these constituents were separated into those produced via mechanobiological processes and those produced vis immunological processes with:

$$\text{Eq(1) } \rho^{\text{mech}}(s) = \int_0^s m_h^{\text{mech}} \left(1 + \Upsilon^{\text{mech}}(\tau)\right)(1 - \exp(-\tau))q^{\text{mech}}(s,\tau)d\tau$$

and

$$\text{Eq(2) } \rho^{\text{infl}}(s) = \int_0^s m_h^{\text{infl}} \left(\Upsilon^{\text{infl}}(\tau)\right)(1 - \exp(-\tau))q^{\text{infl}}(s,\tau)d\tau$$

respectively. For each constituent type, m_h^{infl} and m_h^{mech} are the basal production rates, $\Upsilon^{\text{infl}}(\tau)$ and $\Upsilon^{\text{mech}}(\tau)$ are the time-dependent gain functions, and q^{infl} and q^{mech} track the survival fraction of material produced at past time τ that remains at current time s. Specific functional forms and parameter values for the gain functions and survival functions were the same as those used previously [66]. Constituent deformations were tracked from their constituent-specific stress-free natural configurations into the current equilibrated state via a multiplicative combination of deformations. Mechanical equilibrium was ensured at each time step to identify the evolving loaded geometry of the TEVG.

Case studies were performed that modified the kinetics for both the immuno- and mechano-mediated constituents. We simulated 4 cases: the gain for mechano-mediated production was set to zero $\Upsilon^{\mathrm{mech}}(\tau) = 0$, the gain for immuno-mediated production was set to zero $\Upsilon^{\mathrm{infl}}(\tau) = 0$, and the mechano-mediated constituents were not considered $\rho^{\mathrm{mech}}(s) = 0$.

4.2 Accelerated Degradation

TEVG samples were evaluated for degradation kinetics through accelerated degradation testing in heated PBSs. Rings of 5mm length were cut from 16mm diameter TEVGs, and dry weight was taken. Samples were then submerged in 1x PBS heated to 70C for set time periods before removal. After degradation, samples were washed twice with ddH_2O, frozen to -80C, and lyophilized overnight before measuring the remaining mass. Zero-day control specimens were submerged in PBS for 5 minutes before washing and lyophilization to account for any swelling changes during processing. Samples were then separated into mechanical testing specimens, microstructure specimens, and polymer composition specimens.

Mechanical testing of degraded ring samples was performed on a 100 Series TestResources MTI. Testing was performed with a 10N load cell at a tensile rate of 3mm per second. Tensile load was equated to equivalent pressure through the equation: P = m*g / (2* Z * r), where P = pressure, m = hanging mass, g = gravity, Z = initial axial length of sample, and r = initial internal radius of sample. Burst pressure was defined by the equated pressure which caused sample failure, or defined as 0 mmHg for samples which did not have enough structural integrity to load into the tester, or >1000 mmHg for samples which did not break under the maximum force of the load cell (equivalent to 1000 mmHg).

Microstructure specimens were cut into 5mmx5mm samples and mounted onto SEM mounts with carbon tape. A subset of these samples then had the outer PCLA sponge surface removed using forceps under a dissecting microscope to reveal the inner PGA fiber layer. Samples were sputter coated with gold under argon vacuum to 3nm, and imaged on a Hitachi S4800 SEM at 5kV and 10mA. SEM images were analyzed with FIJI image analysis software. Pore size was calculated by 7 SEM images at 100x of sample lumens. Fiber diameter was calculated by an average of at least 5 PGA fibers.

Following degradation testing, samples of the rings were cut and dissolved at 1mg/mL in 50mM NaOH for 48 hours at 80C to ensure complete degradation of remaining polymer. Aliquots of dissolved solutions were then diluted 1/10 in 50mM NaOH and separately analyzed for lactate, a degradation product of PCLA, and glycolic acid, the degradation product of PGA. Lactate was measured using a commercially available Lactate Assay (Sigma-Aldrich, MO, USA). Glycolic acid was analyzed using a method adapted from Takahashi, 1972 [214]. 50uL of each sample was incubated in 1mL of 0.02% 2,7-dihydroxynapthalene in concentrated sulfuric acid for 20 minutes at 100C. 100uL aliquots were then added to a 96 well plate in duplicate and absorbance was measured at 540nm. Mixed ratios of dissolved pure PCLA and pure PGA were used to generate standard curves.

4.3 Sheep Implantation and Follow-Up

4.3.1 Study design

The objective of this study was to quantify the natural history of neotissue formation and thus neovessel development over 1 year in an established IVC interposition TEVG model [192, 215, 216]. Seeded TEVGs were implanted in 53 lambs, and *in vivo* data were collected via serial angiography and intravascular ultrasound at 1 week, 6 weeks, 6 months, 1 year, two years, and three years [216]. The 1 week time is used for baseline anatomic information; it provides comparable data to the immediate post-operative period, but allows the animal to recover from the initial surgical insult and decreases risks associated with a prolonged anesthesia needed to perform the implantation surgery and an initial catheterization during the same period. The primary endpoint was the narrowest cross-sectional area of the graft on IVUS imaging at each time. No data were excluded from the study.

4.3.2 Bone marrow aspiration, assembly, and implantation of the TEVG

53 lambs underwent bone marrow aspiration (5 mL/kg body weight) and implantation of an autologous cell-seeded TEVG as an intrathoracic IVC interposition graft. Animals were anesthetized using propofol (5 mg/kg) for induction and isoflurane (1-4%) or propofol (20-40 mg/kg/hr) for maintenance. Lambs were placed in the lateral recumbent position, and the area overlying the iliac crest was shaved and prepped in standard sterile fashion. A 5-mm incision was made and an aspiration needle was inserted into the bone. Heparinized syringes (20 mL, 100 U/mL) were used to aspirate bone marrow. Following aspiration, the bone marrow was processed using Ficoll density gradient centrifugation to isolate the bone

marrow-derived mononuclear cells as previously described [217]. Briefly, bone marrow was filtered through 100 μm cell strainers to remove bone spicules and clots. A 1:1 dilution was achieved with phosphate buffered saline (PBS) and the bone marrow was layered onto Ficoll 1077 (Sigma-Aldrich). The plasma and mononuclear cell layers were isolated after centrifugation. The mononuclear cell layer underwent two washes with PBS to yield a cell pellet that was diluted in 20 mL of PBS. Mononuclear cells were vacuum-seeded onto the scaffold which was incubated in autologous plasma until the time of implantation.

4.3.3 Cell characterization and seeding efficiency

After density centrifugation in Ficoll, the bone marrow derived mononuclear cells were diluted 1:100 in 1X PBS then mixed 1:1 with trypan blue to label non-viable cells. Counting was performed manually using a hemocytometer. Viability was determined using trypan blue exclusion. The number of bone marrow-derived mononuclear cells seeded onto a scaffold was quantified as the difference in the total number of cells in the Ficoll-enriched bone marrowderived mononuclear cell solution before and after vacuum-seeding. Dividing this difference in cell number by the surface area of the scaffold provided the average cell density on the scaffold. **Surgery** The scaffolds were implanted in the intrathoracic IVC as previously described [192, 215, 216]. Lambs were placed in a left lateral recumbent position. Depending on each animal's anatomy, a right thoracotomy was made in the fifth or sixth intercostal space, and the thoracic IVC was dissected between the diaphragm and right atrium. A cavoatrial shunt was placed to maintain perfusion during cross-clamping of the IVC. The vessel was clamped and a 2 nonabsorbable monofilament suture. No native vessel was removed. Titanium vascular clips were applied to the suture tails to mark the anastomoses for postoperative imaging. The chest wall, overlying muscle, and skin layers were reapproximated with absorbable sutures.

4.3.4 Interventional imaging

Postoperative catheterizations were performed at 1 week, 6 weeks, 6 months, 1 year, 2 years, and 3 years. Additional imaging was performed as needed based on the animals' clinical conditions. After sedation and intubation, lambs were placed in a left lateral recumbent position. The right internal jugular vein was cannulated and a 9-French sheath (Terumo) was inserted followed by an intravenous bolus of heparin (150 U/kg). A 5 French JR 2.5 catheter (Cook Medical) was passed into the right internal jugular vein through the SVC and into the right atrium. Using an angled Glidewire (Terumo), the JR catheter was then passed through the TEVG into the intraabdominal IVC where a Rosen exchange guidewire (Cook Medical) was placed. The JR catheter was then exchanged for a 5 French multi-track angiographic catheter (NuMed), which was used to measure hemodynamic pressures in the intraabdominal IVC, intrathoracic IVC below and above the TEVG, and within the TEVG. A mean pressure gradient was calculated by subtracting the mean pressure above the TEVG from the mean pressure below the TEVG. A digital angiogram was then obtained by injecting ioversol 68% (Mallinckrodt Pharmaceuticals) through the multitrack angiographic catheter positioned in the intraabdominal IVC. Diameters were measured at seven points: the intraabdominal IVC, low intrathoracic IVC (on the diaphragmatic side of the TEVG), proximal anastomosis (defined with respect to blood flow), midgraft, distal anastomosis, high intrathoracic IVC (on the atrial side of the TEVG), and the area of most severe narrowing. The proximal and distal anastomoses were identified by the aforementioned surgically-placed radiopaque clips. A 0.035-inch digital intravascular ultrasound catheter (Volcano) was advanced through the graft over the Rosen guidewire to obtain images at the same seven points measured during angiography. These images were analyzed using Volcano software to obtain a cross-sectional area as described previously [216]. Neotissue deposition within the TEVG was measured using IVUS. Graphical reconstructions of IVUS imaging data were performed using Rhino 3D.

4.3.5 Euthanasia

At the prescribed endpoint, animals were deeply sedated with ketamine (20 mg/kg) and diazepam (0.02-0.08 mg/kg), followed by induction of bilateral pneumothoraces and exsanguination. A complete veterinary necropsy was performed at the time of TEVG explantation. Animals were also euthanized if they developed critical stenosis (n = 2), defined here as graft narrowing with systemic symptoms. Animals that were not euthanized for critical stenosis were euthanized at 6 weeks (n=11) 6 months (n=10) or 12 months (n=12) post implantation. The remaining animals were survived for long-term follow up, with n=3 euthanized at 18 months for late-term mechanical testing.

5.4 Construction of 3D TEVG Geometries

3D CT angiography data was collected at some of 1, 6, 26, 52, and 104 week timepoints after graft implantation for each of 40 animals. 1 of 40 animals were sacrificed after the 6 week imaging, 11 after 26 weeks, 14 after 52 weeks, and 14 animals were followed through the 104 week timepoint. TEVG boundaries were defined using radiopaque markers at distal and proximal anastomoses that remained visible throughout the duration of the imaging study. Reconstruction of the TEVG within the borders defined by the radiopaque markers was performed in an opensource software (Simvascular, www.simtk.org). The imaging data were used to reconstruct the 3D TEVG geometry through an image segmentation technique and the final 3D TEVG geometry was discretized and exported to an opensource data analysis and visualization software (Paraview, www.paraview.org). The volumes of the 3D TEVG geometries were attained and average volume was computed for each timepoint.

5.5 Magnetic Resonance Imaging

Animals were evaluated at 1 week, 6 weeks and 1 year post implantation with black blood TSE MRI, contrast enhanced 3D radial MR angiography (MRA), MR 2D and 3D flow velocity mapping, and delayed enhancement imaging for fibrosis. Animals were sedated with propofol and intubated for all MRI imaging studies. Imaging was performed on a Siemans 3T Prisma MRI scanner. In each subject, native IVC proximal and distal to the graft, proximal and distal graft anastomotic sites, and the mid graft were analyzed and compared between 1 week, 6 weeks, and 1year. Patterns of luminal distortion were assessed, and characterized using flow velocity changes, and tissue response as demonstrated on dynamic early contrast enhancement (DCE), and delayed enhancement (DE).

4.6 *Ex Vivo* Mechanical Testing

The TEVGs were excised with the adjacent thoracic inferior vena cava. The perivascular tissue was gently cleaned and the composite vessel-graft construct was mounted on custom made plastic cannulas in Hanks buffered solution. The composite construct was secured to the cannula at the atrium and the diaphragm junctions using 3-0 sutures. Tubular biaxial testing was performed using a computer-controlled device[218]. Force and pressure were measured using standard transducers, diameter was tracked with an optical video-scope and length was prescribed using a stepper motor. The vessel was initially equilibrated at ~5mmHg and preconditioned with six cycles of pressurization from 0-30mmHg, at *in vivo* stretch; *in vivo* stretch is the stretch at which axial force is approximately a constant with change in pressure. The biaxial protocol has a total of seven tests, three pressure-inflation tests (1-30mmHg) at constant axial stretches and four axial force-extension tests at constant pressures, details of which can be found elsewhere[66]. Pressure-diameter and circumferential stress-stretch behaviors from the pressure-distension test at *in vivo* stretch are reported for the 6 week and 18 month samples and the native inferior vena cava.

4.7 Vasoreactivity Testing

TEVG, adjacent thoracic IVC, and native thoracic IVC (n=4 per group), just inferior to the graft, were dissected from the same lamb and placed in ice-cold Krebs buffer containing (mM): NaCl, 118; KCl, 4.7; KH_2PO_4, 1.18; $MgSO_4 \cdot 7H_2O$, 1.64; $NaHCO_3$, 25.0; Glucose, 5.55; Na-Pyruvate, 2.0; $CaCl_2 \cdot 2H_2O$, 2.52; (pH=7.4). The vessels were cut into ~5-mm rings and mounted in a tissue bath system (Radnoti LLC, Covina, CA) containing 15 mL

Krebs (37°C – 95:5% O_2:CO_2) at 0.5 g of resting tension. Force was acquired using isometric force transducers (Radnoti) connected to a PowerLab 16/30 (AD Instruments, Colorado Springs, Colorado). Data were recorded using LabChart 7 (AD Instruments). After a one hour equilibration period, the viability of the vessels was tested using 60 mM KCl. Following washing and a return to baseline tension, the vessels were pre-constricted with 1 nM endothelin-1 (ET-1, Sigma-Aldrich, St. Louis, MO).[219] Following pre-constriction, endothelial-dependent and endothelium-independent relaxation was assessed by adding increasing concentrations (10^{-9} M to 10^{-4} M) of acetylcholine (ACh, Sigma) and sodium nitroprusside (SNP, Sigma), respectively. After testing vessel dilatory capacity, the vessels were then subjected to cumulative concentrations of ET-1 (10^{-12} M to 10^{-8} M) to assess their ability to contract. Relaxation responses were plotted as a percentage of the ET-1 induced contraction for each vessel, and contraction to ET-1 was plotted as a percentage of the maximal response to 60 mM KCl. Concentration response data were fit to a log function, and log EC_{50} values were calculated by nonlinear regression analysis using GraphPad Prism 7.0 software (GraphPad, La Jolla, CA). The pharmacologically tested samples were imaged under SEM as well as en face immunofluorescent staining with CD31 and eNOS to evaluate the endothelial cells lining the lumen of the neovessel.

4.8 Histology

TEVGs and adjacent IVC tissue was explanted, fixed with 4% formalin for 1 week, then transferred to 70% ethanol for long-term storage. Upon removal from ethanol, tissues were cut into smaller pieces to facilitate paraffin embedding and enable histological sections to be prepared within the proximal IVC, the TEVG near the proximal anastomosis, mid-graft, and near the distal anastomosis, as well as within the distal IVC. 4-µm transverse sections were mounted on slides and heat fixed. Standard techniques were adopted for hematoxylin and eosin, Picro-Sirius Red, Masson's Trichrome, Movat Pentachrome, and Hart's Elastin staining. Immunohistochemistry was used to detect the antigens of interest. Samples underwent heat-induced antigen retrieval with Dako target retrieval solution in a pressure cooker using either citrate buffer (pH 6.0) or Tris-EDTA buffer (pH 9.0) followed by blocking for endogenous peroxidase (3.0% $H2O2$ in $H2O$) and non-specific binding (3% normal goat serum in Background Sniper, BioCare Medical). After primary antibody incubation overnight at 4C, sections were incubated sequentially in appropriate biotinylated secondary antibodies (1:1500, Vector) and streptavidin-horseradish peroxidase (Vector). DAB+ substrate chromogen (Vector) was used for color development. All samples were counterstained with Gill's hematoxylin (Vector) prior to dehydration and cover-slipping.

Histomorphometric analysis of stenosis was performed in imageJ (NIH, Bethesda< Maryland). Boundaries between the neoadventitia and the outer surface of the scaffold, between the inner surface of the scaffold and the neointima, as well as the luminal surface were traced. Area and perimeter values for these boundary lines were used to calculate the luminal area remaining as compared to a scaffold at implantation, neointimal area, and the fold-increase in scaffold cross-sectional area. These values were then used to estimate factors that contribute to overall stenosis including Intramural growth and inward remodeling.

4.9 Statistical Analysis

Statistical analyses and linear regressions were performed, and graphs were created using GraphPad Prism version 7.03 (GraphPad Software Inc.). Groups were compared using t-tests, except in cases of unequal variances, where nonparametric Mann-Whitney tests were performed. Linear regressions were performed utilizing histological staining as independent variable, with histomorphometric measures of intramural growth and inward remodeling on identical animals as dependent variable. p value of 0.05 was considered significant.

5. Figures

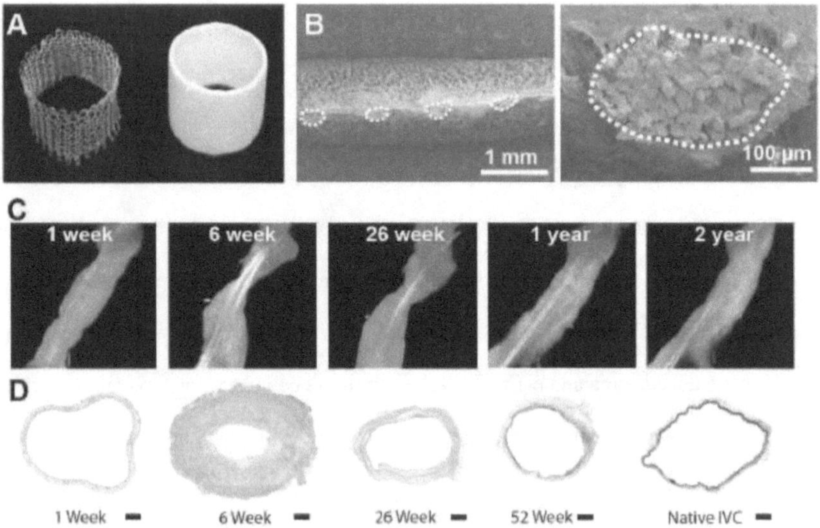

Figure 4-1Natural History of Tissue Engineered Vascular Graft Development

A) TEVG created from PGA mesh (left) coated in an inner and outer sponge of PCLA (right). B) Magnified SEM of TEVG demonstrating sponge layers of PCLA with PGA fibers outlines with white. C) Representative 3D reconstructions of angiographic images of TEVGs over 2 years following implantation in a sheep model. D) Representative histology changes in TEVG demonstrate characteristic changes becoming similar to IVC after 1 year *in vivo*. Scale bar = 100 μm.

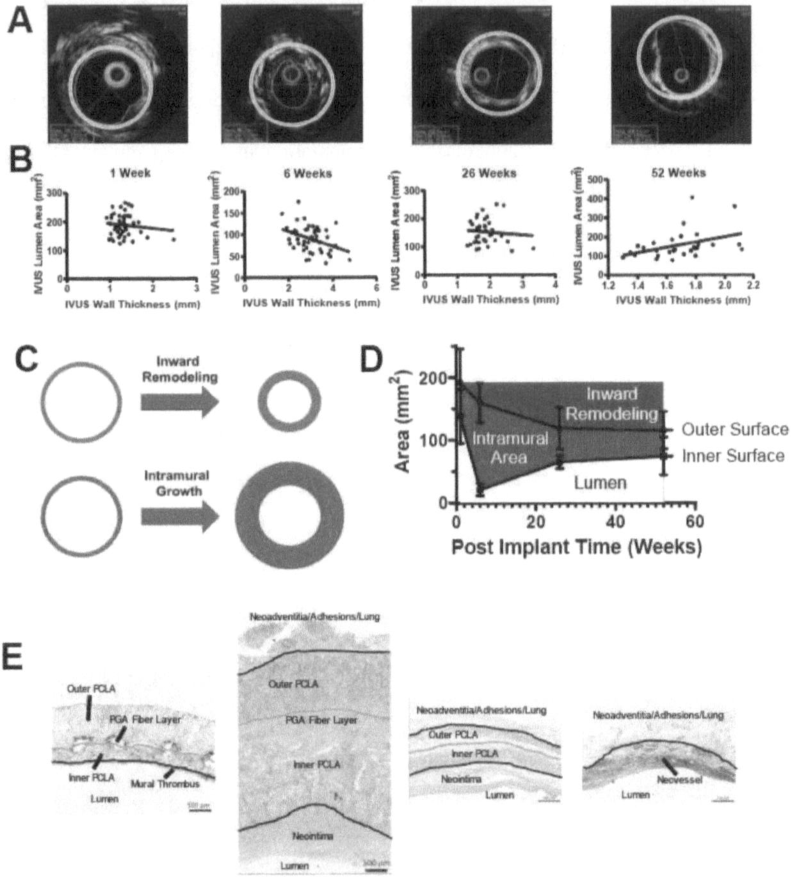

Figure 4-2 Histomorphometric Changes During Neotissue Formation and Development

A) Intravascular ultrasound (IVUS) imaging of TEVG, with lumen outlined in green and original TEVG size shown in yellow. Quantification of wall thickness and lumen area shown in (B). C) Remodeling in TEVGs occurs through two main processes, inward remodeling (blue) with a decrease of outer diameter, and intramural growth (red) with a thickening of the vessel wall. D) Quantification of changes in inner and outer diameter of TEVGs in the sheep model. E) Close up representative trichrome staining demonstrating intramural growth, neointima formation, and subsequent scaffold thinning and degradation in creation of a neovessel.

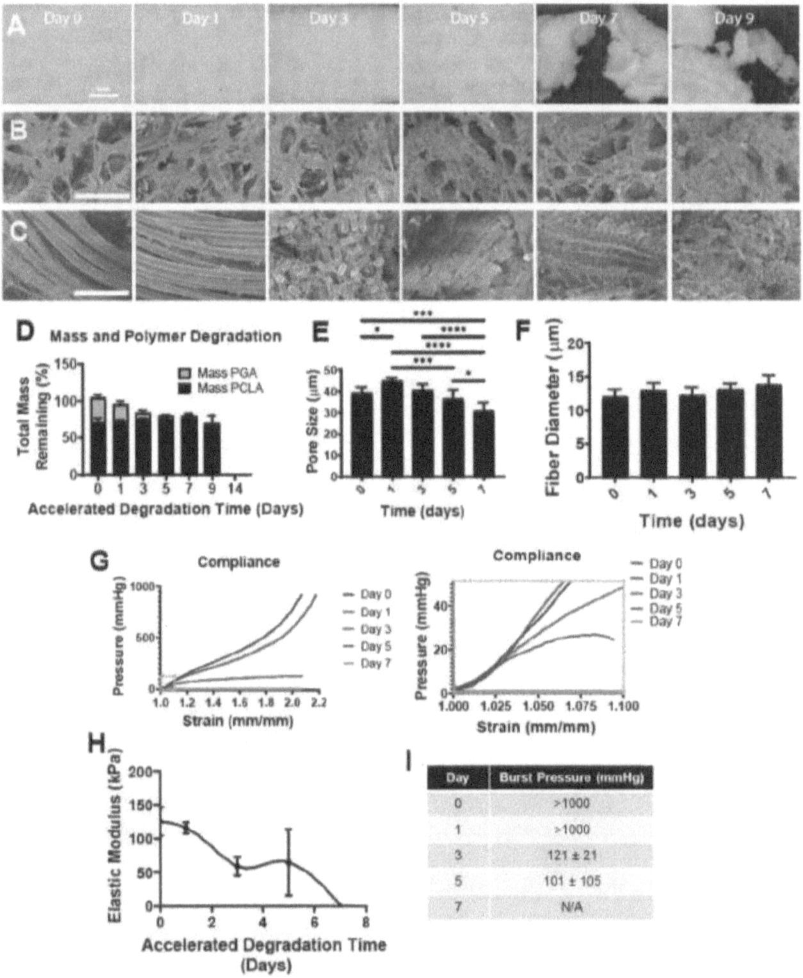

Figure 4-3 In Vitro Accelerated Degradation of TEVG Scaffolds

Accelerated degradation studies of TEVG demonstrates a breaking down of the macrostructure (A) as well as the PCLA (B) and PGA (C) microstructures. D) Mass and polymer degradation of TEVGs, with PCLA pore (E) and fiber (F) sizes quantified. G) Strain vs pressure curves of mechanical testing of TEVGs subjected to accelerated degradation studies, with blue-outlined low pressure region magnified on right. Changes in elastic modulus (H) and burst pressure (I) quantified from mechanical testing. Scale bars A) 1 mm, B&C) 100 μm.

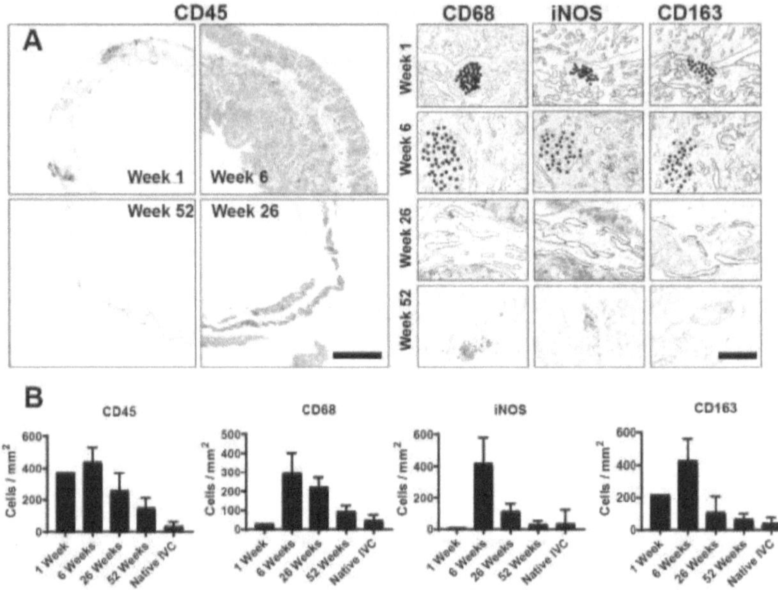

Figure 4-4 Inflammatory Constituents Throughout Neovessel Formation

A) Representative histology of inflammatory cells, including CD45, CD68, iNOS, and CD163 over 1 year implantation. PGA labeled in solid black, with PCLA outlined in black. B) quantifications of histological inflammatory markers. Scale bars left) 2000 μm, right) 200 μm.

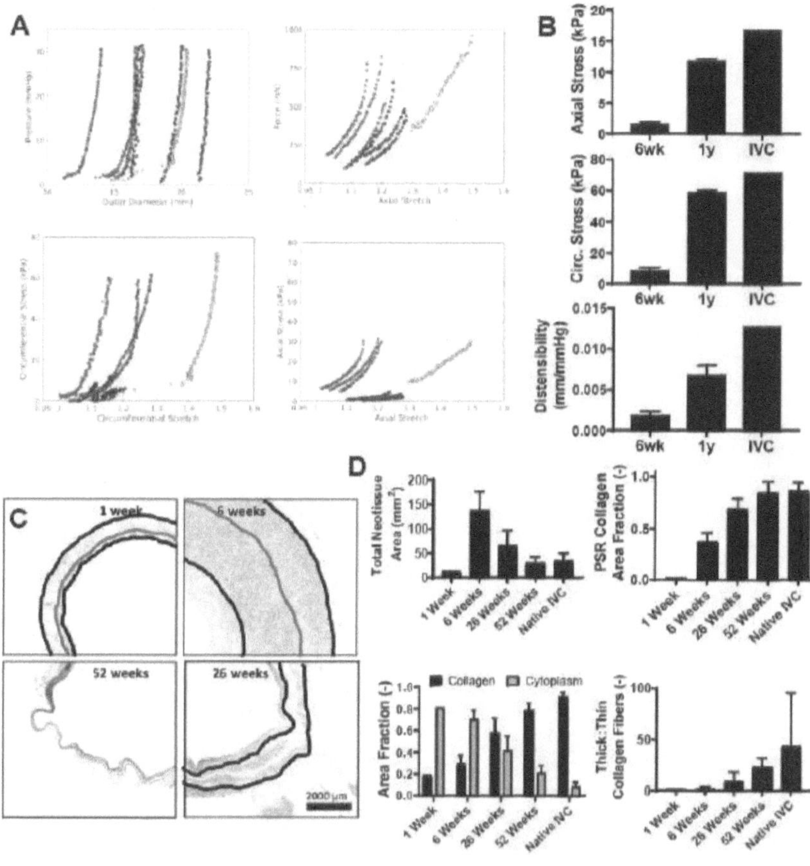

Figure 4-5 Mechanical Constituents Throughout Neovessel Formation

A) Representative *ex vivo* biaxial mechanical testing of TEVGs at 6 weeks and 1.5 years as well as native IVC. Mechanical measurements from biaxial mechanical testing shown in (B). C) Representative trichrome staining of TEVGs demonstrating changes in thickness as well as ECM and cellular make-up of neotissue. PCLA outlined in black, with PGA layer noted in blue. D) Quantifications of trichrome and picrosirius red staining.

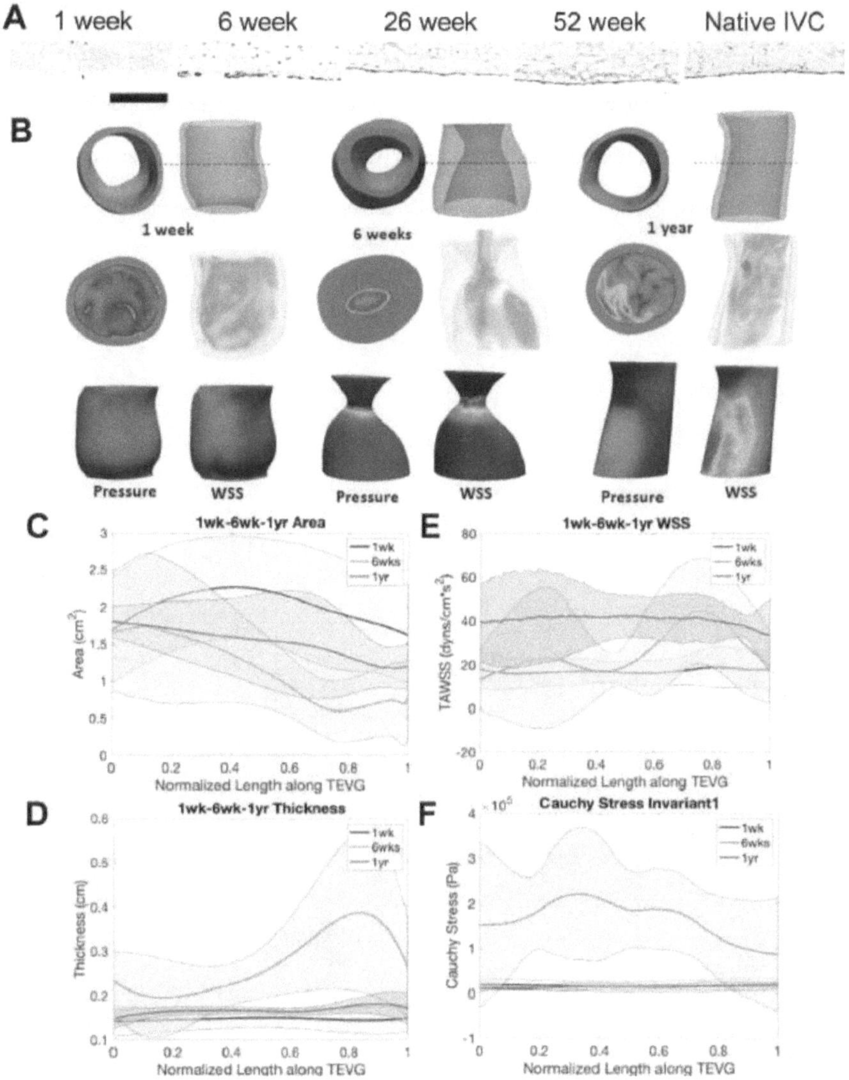

Figure 4-6 Characterization of Fluid Flow in TEVGs

A) eNOS staining of TEVG neotissue and native IVC lumens, demonstrating the development of continuous endothelial layer by 6 months. Scale bar = 100μm. B) 3D reconstructions of TEVGs from computational fluid dynamics modeling using MRI data. Average ± standard deviation of area (C), thickness (D), wall shear stress (E), and Cauchy Stress (F) shown along the normalized length of the graft for each time point.

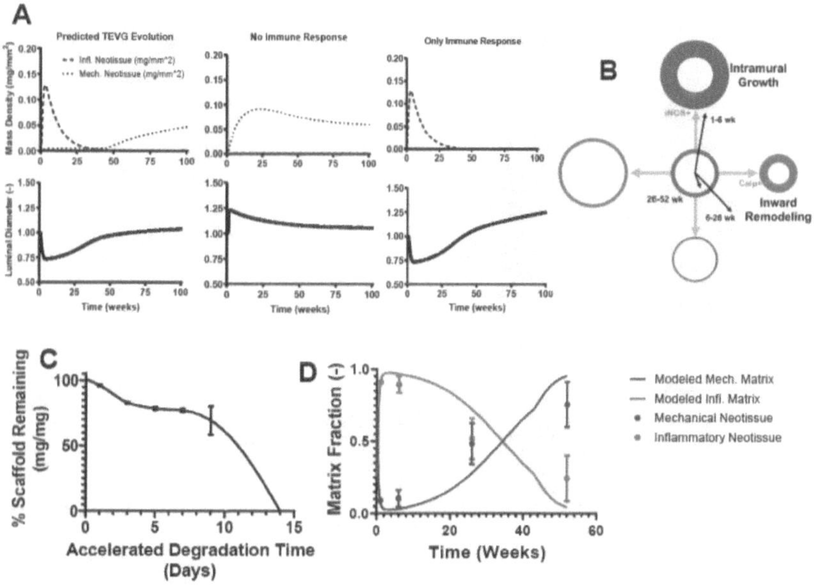

Figure 4-7 Mathematical Model predicts TEVG Neovessel Formation

A) Mathematical modeling of TEVG neotissue formation, demonstrating the combinatory effects of inflammation and mechanomediated neotissue formation and remodeling (left). Computational modeling result of neotissue formation and remodeling in the absence of an immune response (middle). Computational modeling result of neotissue formation and remodeling in absence of mechano-mediated response (right). B) Plot of inward remodeling vs intramural growth, with changes over time demonstrated by arrows from the origin. C) Accelerated degradation mass of TEVG over time. D) Comparison of computational modeling prediction of inflammatory and mechanical neotissue to histological findings.

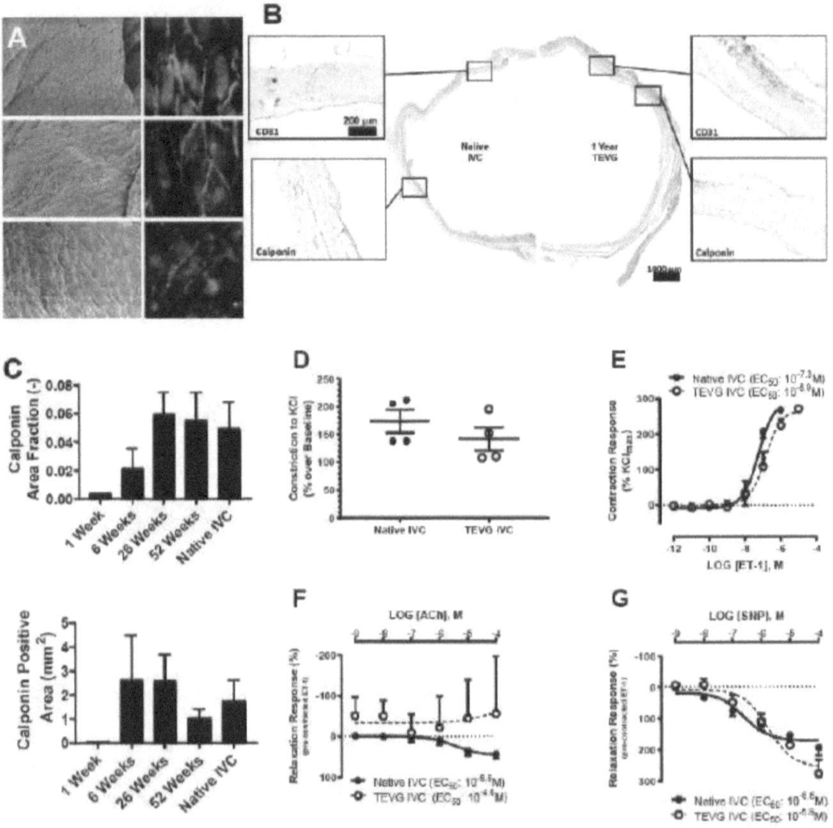

Figure 4-8 TEVGs develop into Neovessels with Native Structure and Vasoactivity

A) SEM (left) and *en face* staining (right) of explanted TEVG neovessel luminal surface demonstrates confluent layer of endothelial cells. CD31 marked with green and eNOS in red. B) Representative H&E histology of native IVC (left) to 1 year TEVG (right), with insets showing CD31-lined lumen (top) and layers of calponin-positive smooth muscle cells (bottom). C) Quantification of calponin staining from explanted TEVGs. Results of vasoreactivity testing of TEVGS implanted for over 1.5 years and adjacent native IVC, demonstrating comparable responses to KCL (D), Endothelin-1 (E), Acetylcholine (F), and Sodium Nitroprusside (G).

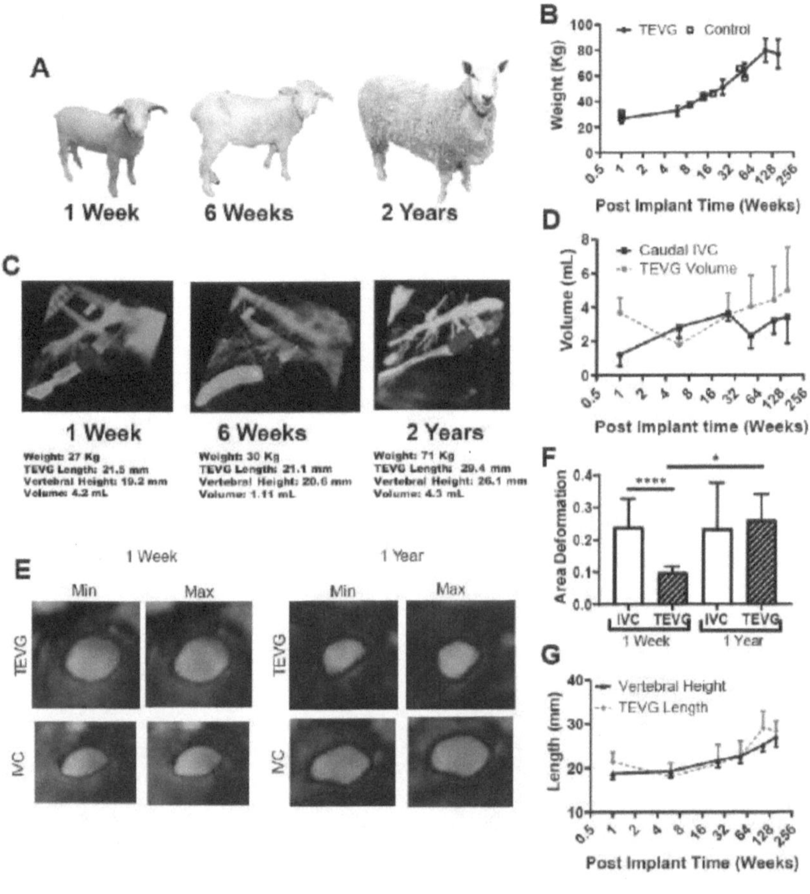

Figure 4-9 TEVG Neovessels Demonstrate Biological Growth

A) Representative images of growth of sheep over implantation time. B) Quantification of weight for TEVG-implanted and non-implanted control animals over long term implantation. C) Representative 3D angiography imaging of a sheep over the implantation time. Native IVC colored yellow, TEVG colored dark blue, and surrounding anatomic structures colored light blue. Measurements taken from each representative image shown below. D) Quantification of TEVG volume compared to caudal IVS of the same animals. E) Representative images of midgraft TEVG at minimum and maximum area over a cardiac cycle as measured by MRI, at 1 week (Left) and 1 year (Right). F) Quantification of area deformation of TEVG and adjacent IVC at 1 week and 1 year post-implantation. G) Length of TEVG and vertebral body as measured from angiography. Red boxes denote the time until complete TEVG degradation.

Chapter 5. Conclusions and Future Directions

1. Overview

In this book, I have explored the mechanisms guiding neotissue formation and remodeling from several avenues, in order to better isolate the independent effects of each stimulus. Scaffold biomechanics, as measured using an aortic murine model, had an effect at altering failure modes as well as the make-up of developed neotissue. Host biology, as measured using venous TEVG murine model, was shown to have strong effects, particularly in how males and females differ in terms of neotissue formation. Finally, we examined the effects of long term implantation in a large animal model, demonstrating that over long implantation times the TEVG develops into a functional neovessel with native-like architecture and functions, including vasoreactivity and growth potential.

2. Summary of Findings

2.1 Mechanical

Braided small-diameter arterial grafts of PGA with and without PGS coating were manufactured at the edges of the braidable parameter space and evaluated for failure mode and performance within a murine infrarenal aortic implantation model. We demonstrated that braiding parameters, and the resulting physical properties of the scaffolds, had a substantial effect on the failure mode (bleeding, early rupture, late rupture) *in vivo*. Creating too loose of a braid led to early failure following implantation, while creating an exceedingly tight braid created stress shielding that hindered neotissue formation, resulting in aneurysmal failure of the graft when the scaffold lost mechanical integrity. Braiding parameters and the anti-inflammatory PGS coating also affected the histological make-up of the resulting neovessels. This work also demonstrated that detailed ultrasound analysis and explant biaxial testing allow for the longitudinal *in vivo* evaluation of morphometric properties.

The application of statistical regression analysis on the neotissue formation outcomes allowed us to highlight potential mechanisms at play between scaffold architecture and the developed neotissue. Increasing the circumferential stiffness of the TEAGs, through increasing the PPSI or the braiding angle, resulted in increased collagen deposition, but decreased elastin and decreased distensilbility at 12 weeks. A positive correlation was also found between CD68 and calponin staining, suggesting that the inflammation triggered by the scaffold had a downstream effect on the infiltration of smooth muscle cells.

2.2 Biological

Utilizing a murine IVC TEVG model, we have shown multiple effects of sex on a cardiovascular tissue engineering model, as well as sex-specific effects of tamoxifen. Sex-specific differences in untreated mice, particularly in cellularity, deposition of neotissue, development of giant cells in reaction to biomaterial implantation, and differences in rate of biomaterial degradation have strong consequences towards the development of ideal tissue engineering solutions.

Results related to the inflammatory response further this understanding and go on to suggest that macrophages and monocytes of males and females respond differently to implanted biomaterials, an important consideration for evaluation of biomaterials as well as their translation to the clinic. Females created more foreign body giant cells and produced more collagen. Males, on the other hand, degraded the implanted biomaterial much more rapidly despite similar levels of macrophages. The large difference in the inflammatory response between sexes compared to similar M1/M2 ratios seen in this study may suggest that additional factors related to macrophage and monocyte function in response to biomaterials should be investigated in future studies.

In addition to sex differences in tissue regeneration and remodeling, we showed that tamoxifen treatment alters the host response to TEVGs. Our findings in female mice showed that Ki67-labeled proliferation and CD31-labeled endothelial cell expression were decreased at two weeks in our TEVGs.

Throughout early experiments, the significant weight loss associated with the tamoxifen chow treatment raised concern of weight loss and malnutrition being causal of the findings in this study, as opposed to effects of tamoxifen directly, leading to the use of tamoxifen IP injections. While results between tamoxifen chow or daily tamoxifen IP injection are similar in females, there were several differences noted, mainly in effect size. These differences may be due to differences in bioavailability of tamoxifen for each dosing strategy, or by the differences in dosing between a controlled IP injection and an *ad libitum* diet of tamoxifen chow. In addition, there is the possibility that the weight loss seen in the tamoxifen chow group exhibited additional effects on top of the tamoxifen itself, potentiating some effects and antagonizing others.

Overall, this study demonstrated the complicated biological mechanisms at play in tissue engineering constructs. Even in syngeneic animals, the effects of sex cannot be ignored, and in fact can provide insight into important biological differences and potential avenues to improve tissue engineering outcomes. The use of any treatment on an animal or patient, in this case tamoxifen, can also have many unanticipated off-target effects on a tissue engineering system. The dosing route of the drug may also be an important factor in determining any confounding effects. Careful development of experimental design and thoughtful analysis of resulting outcomes will be crucial for the continued development of the field of tissue engineering, and determination of the biological mechanisms at play.

2.3 Long Term implantation

Utilizing a large animal model provides two important advantages over the small animal models used in previous chapters. First, the large animal model provides the opportunity to evaluate the TEVG in an environment that more closely resembles the clinical intended formulation, with more appropriate size, mechanical forces, and fluid dynamic properties. Second, the longer lifespan of the sheep allows for longer term evaluation of the TEVG, past the point of complete scaffold degradation, to evaluate the long term remodeling and outcomes of the TEVG.

Though the early time period after implantation is dominated by inflammatory cues from the scaffold, at longer times the native processes that govern vascular behavior mediate the structural changes. By considering these interacting phases of neovessel formation, we hypothesized that the neovessel could approach the structural and functional features of a native vessel after long term implantation. These results reinforce that two distinct phases of TEVG remodeling aid in the formation of a functional graft, an early neotissue formation phase and a later neovessel remodeling phase. Furthermore, the importance of the native mechanobiological processes to prevent late stenosis or dilatation was evident. As such, native cues for blood vessel growth and remodeling within the body were suggested to take over within the neovessel, which could generate a vessel with a cellular and ECM make-up, mechanical properties, and biological reactivity similar to native blood vessels. We therefore examined the evolution of our TEVGs through long term implantation studies to examine the potential for the emergence of functional neovessel.

In vitro accelerated degradation testing allowed the analysis of scaffold properties over degradation time without implantation. While the TEVG degrades, the mechanical cues within the neotissue change dramatically. In the very early time points, the load within the wall of the TEVG is carried only by the polymer scaffold, which stress-shields the inflammatory cells and the deposited inflammatory matrix. However, over time the scaffold degrades, the inflammatory stimulus subsides, degradation outpaces production, and the mechanical load is shifted to the cells and deposited matrix. This mechanical stimulus allows for reorganization of the neotissue into a more native-like state.

Histological analysis demonstrated a vessel with rapid changes in cellularity and ECM make up over the first several months *in vivo*, followed by more gradual changes over longer time points as the make-up approaches that of the native vessel. These changes are seen in inflammation, smooth muscle cells, collagen amounts and organization, wall thickness, and mechanical properties both *in vivo* and *ex vivo*.

In addition, the time period of cellular and histomorphometric changes corroborated our computational model predictions. The degree of wall thickening due to intramural growth and remodeling seen at 6 weeks *in vivo*, predicted to be due to the inflammatory stimuli of the scaffold, correlated with the inflammatory iNOS+ cell staining within the wall of the graft. Similarly, the inward remodeling and wall thinning, predicted to be driven by mechanical stimuli, was found to be correlated with the presence of calponin+ smooth muscle cells within the wall of the graft.

The *in vivo* growth of the TEVGs within the sheep model further demonstrated the multiple phases of remodeling. During the early neotissue formation phase, the TEVG expanded in wall thickness, limiting the lumen area as well as contracting axially. However, after the graft lost mechanical integrity through degradation and the inflammatory stimulus subsided, the TEVG entered the neovessel remodeling phase, growing in both length and diameter at similar rates to the surrounding native vasculature.

Overall, this work demonstrates the potential of tissue engineering in creating tissues that not only resemble the architecture of the tissues they are replacing, but also the biological functionality and long term status indistinguishable from that of the original native structures. This finding has important clinical implications for TEVGs, particularly those involved in our previous and current clinical trials of the TEVG in the Fontan circulation. In the early months post-implantation we can expect the TEVG to remodel rapidly, although not directly following native growth and remodeling cues. In this neotissue formation stage the clinical evaluation of these TEVGs should focus on prevention of symptomatic stenosis or overgrowth of neotissue. As time progresses and the neotissue formation phase is replaced with the neovessel remodeling phase, the clinical following of the TEVG can be treated as any other vein within the body, as it approaches the structure and function of the native blood vessel over time following native stimuli.

3. Implications for Cardiovascular Tissue Engineering

This work has demonstrated the multitude of interconnected mechanisms at play throughout TEVG neotissue formation and remodeling. Detailed understanding of the biological and mechanical forces at play, as well as their dynamic changes over the implantation time, is crucial to the rational design of tissue engineering devices with optimal outcomes at early and late time points. Due to the difficult nature of isolating individual mechanisms in the complicated web of pathways present in any biological system, computational modeling has a key role to play in the future of rational design.

An important benefit to our computational-experimental approach used in these studies and throughout our laboratory work is the ability for computational studies to guide relevant experimentation, and the ability of experimental results to update and refine the computational model. As the material and mechanical properties of the scaffold are the guiding forces of inflammation and neotissue formation in the early time points, computational modeling can be beneficial in navigating the potential scaffold parameter space *in silico* [25]. Coupled with guided *in vivo* experimentation around the edges of this parameter space, this computational-experimental approach can suggest key time points and scaffolding parameters for evaluation, and experimental results can be compared and contrasted with modeling outcomes to determine new effects and interactions to create a more accurate model [26-28]. This method has the benefit of decreasing the needed number of animals for experimentation, and may accelerate new design development through the suggestion of optimized scaffold parameters.

While the outcomes of these studies have direct implication to the development of tissue engineered vascular grafts, the techniques and findings in these book also hold relevance to other areas of tissue engineering, particularly cardiovascular tissue engineering. TEVGs have had the most successful development and implementation to the clinic of the cardiovascular tissue engineering devices, but tissue engineered heart valves (TEHV) and cardiac patches have also been in development and seen successes in the benchtop and clinic.

As with other tissue engineering areas, many TEHV developments up until recently have been done in an empiric manner, with investigative hunches being used to improve designs and experiment to find more successful outcomes [160]. However, more recent studies have shown great success in taking a more rational design approach to tissue engineering. Combining in-depth mathematical modeling with carefully designed experiments, the unknown mechanisms guiding tissue formation can be better elucidated. This advanced understanding can then be used to develop grafts with more ideal properties to lead to better outcomes for neotissue formation and performance over the short and long term. By combining computational modeling with a sheep model of transcatheter valve replacement, a sheep tissue engineered pulmonary valve was delivered on a stent and followed for 1 year

[220]. Explanted tissue showed strong agreement with predicted remodeling. The continued integration of computational modeling with tissue engineering areas, coupled with careful mechanistic experimental design, will likely be fruitful in developing a new generation of tissue engineering devices, including TEVGs, TEHVs, and cardiac patches with ideal performance in the short and long term.

4. Future Directions

The work described in this book opens many avenues for future directions of scientific exploration. The use of braiding to control neotissue formation through mechanical signals could be expanded upon through detailed timecourse explants and histological and biomechanical analysis, in order to determine the timescales associated with the differences in neotissue formation, as well as extending the total implantation time longer to determine if the effects on neotissue in the early time frame affect long term neovessel outcomes. In addition, more detailed biomechanical evaluation, including the use of collagenase and elastase, could aid in determining if and when the mechanical components of the neotissue ECM become functional and mature.[221]

The biological experiments demonstrated differences between male and female mice, and the use of tamoxifen suggests that these affects may be due to hormonal differences between the sexes. These results provide a new avenue into determining the effects of hormonal differences in wound healing as well as tissue engineering. As hormones can be modulated by a number of natural and artificial phenomena, including sex, age, disease state, or exogenous hormone use, several evaluations could be undertaken to gain insight into potential differences between tissue engineering devices designed for children vs adults, or the effects of hormone therapy at improving/hindering tissue engineering outcomes.[222]

Long term implantation studies of TEVG neovessel formation and remodeling demonstrated that TEVGS are capable of becoming functional neovessels after a year *in vivo*. However, the timeline of vasoreactivity development remains to be determined, and could be examined in future studies. In addition, the evaluation of new, computational modeling-driven TEVG designs could be evaluated within the large animal model in order to refine model parameters as well as determine potential clinically relevant outcomes prior to human implantations.

In order to design and translate tissue engineering products to the clinic, more detailed understanding of the mechanisms involved in neotissue formation and remodeling are required. There is a large benefit of utilizing translational research in tissue engineering, comparing results and designing appropriate studies between humans, large animals, small animals, and computational models [190, 223]. The rational design of new tissue engineering iterations relies on the development and careful understanding of both large and small animal models. A recently developed model for heart valve and heart valve leaflet transplantation in a mouse allows for mechanistic studies of how TEHVs develop, and the importance of different graft and host characteristics, similar to those techniques described in this book [224].

Improvements in computational modeling coupled with carefully designed animal studies may allow for a more detailed, mechanistic understanding of the pathway from implanted biomaterial to functional neotissue. Computational modeling of the bio-chemo-mechanics of the environment including interactions between cell types, implanted graft parameters, and cytokines allows for the prediction *in silico* of the effect of pharmacologic modifications and interventions on neotissue development [225]. Separately, a model evaluating the effect of changing graft parameters allowed for the prediction of short and long term outcomes of graft design changes, and predicted design parameters based on the preferred long term outcomes [96]. Combining these model-based parameter predictions with current TEVG manufacturing techniques and *in vitro* scaffold testing methods could allow rapid evaluation of potential scaffolds without the immediate need of *in vivo* experimentation.

Rational design and improvement of TEVGs is predicated on the accuracy of the utilized *in vitro* and *in vivo* models. While small animal models are beneficial for syngeneity and the utility of transgenic animal experiments with large group sizes, the physical scale differences between mice and humans can have large effects on a number of important systems, such as cellular migration distance, endothelialization timeline, and fluid dynamics [112, 159]. Large animal models allow for more physiologic length scales, lifetimes, and hemodynamic parameters similar to those seen in clinical patients. However, all animal models have the limitation of not being humans, and can demonstrate varying differences in cellular mechanisms. Because of this, it is important to evaluate all experiments and results in the context of the host species, and determine how these results may be affected by adaptation to human patients. In addition, it is worth noting that the cardiovascular scenario of our grafts is not identical to that encountered in the clinic. In clinical patients, our TEVGs are utilized in the Fontan circuit, connecting the IVC to the pulmonary arties and bypassing the heart [65]. Recent research into creating a survival model of a sheep Fontan procedure may open the door to more clinically relevant animal model experiments [226].

Three-dimensional imaging and analysis have become commonplace in the clinic to evaluate congenital malformations and plan corrective surgeries. Combination of 3D imaging with the rapidly improving field of 3D printing has provided many clinicians with additional tools for diagnosis, management, and education of congenital heart diseases. As these technologies continue to improve and combine with the field of tissue engineering, we are beginning to see the development of patient-specific stents, grafts, and patches [227].

Combination of tissue engineering products with genetic engineering approaches may allow for improving tissue engineering approaches, however much study still remains in both of these areas, as well as their effects on each other within a growing patient [228]. In conjunction with this area of research, there is concern that cells from diseased patients may not be suitable for tissue engineering since they are inherently damaged as well [229]. Previous clinical missteps such as those with early tissue engineered products such as tissue engineered heart valves demonstrates the need for regulatory oversight of tissue engineered products to prevent patient morbidity and mortality. However, regulatory strategies become more complicated with tissue engineering devices, as traditional definitions of implanted materials and the testing strategies typically applied to determine suitability do not appropriately predict tissue engineering device effectiveness [230].

5. Concluding Remarks

TEVGs are a promising tool for the future of congenital heart surgery, showing the potential to develop into autologous blood vessels with the ability to grow and respond to native stimuli. However, the mechanisms that guide neotissue formation and remodeling are multifaceted and highly intertwined, making careful experimental design and evaluation of results critical to understanding the mechanisms at play. The future creation of next generation tissue engineering devices with ideal properties and performance relies on the rational design of such products, and a computational-experimental approach has shown promise in improving and accelerating that process. Mechanistic understanding of the roles of scaffold properties, host biological properties such as inflammation, and native growth cues will allow for the development of treatments for not only congenital heart disease, but a multitude of medical ailments requiring augmentation or replacement of tissues.